The Madness That is Also in Us

Eugenio Borgna
Translated by Jamie Richards
and Adrian Nathan West

The Madness That is Also in Us

La follia che è anche in noi

PETER LANG

Bruxelles · Berlin · Chennai · Lausanne · New York · Oxford

Bibliographic information published by the Deutsche Nationalbibliothek.
The German National Library lists this publication in the German National Bibliography;
detailed bibliographic data is available on the Internet at http://dnb.d-nb.de.

Library of Congress Cataloging-in-Publication Data
LCCN: 2025049024

This book has been translated thanks to a grant from the Italian Ministry of Foreign Affairs
and International Cooperation.

Questo libro è stato tradotto grazie a una sovvenzione del Ministero degli Affari Esteri e
della Cooperazione Internazionale italiano.

La follia che è anche in noi
© 2019 Giulio Einaudi editore s.p.a., Torino

ISBN 978-3-0343-5107-2 (Print)
ISBN 978-3-0343-5108-9 (ePDF)
ISBN 978-3-0343-5109-6 (ePub)
DOI 10.3726/b23363
Dépôt légal D/2025/5678/67

© 2026 Peter Lang Group AG, Lausanne, Switzerland
Published by P.I.E. PETER LANG s.a., Brussels (Belgium)

info@peterlang.com

www.peterlang.com

Contents

Preface

Eugenio Borgna is, equally with Franco Basaglia, the most important Italian psychiatrist.

If Basaglia gave psychiatric patients back their freedom (with his reform that led to the passage of Law 180 in Italy in 1978), Borgna gave psychiatry back its soul.

And more: he brought it into conversation with philosophy, literature, sociology, spirituality. He took inspiration from these areas of knowledge to practice a human and humane form of psychiatry: phenomenological in nature (like Franco Basaglia, and to some extent, the psychiatrist and writer Mario Tobino), it asks us to put illness aside in order to approach the afflicted with empathy, a capacity for identification, and an attention to their inner world—not solely to their body (as somatological psychiatry—asylum psychiatry—does, only viewing patients exclusively as bearers of a "diseased organ").

This marvelous book, *The Madness That Is Also in Us*, follows Borgna through sixty years of work (and writing) both within and without the asylum, under the sign of the (ethical) revolution that phenomenology sparked in psychiatry.

The book is divided into four chapters, entitled The Revolution in Psychiatry, The Psychiatry of Yesterday, The Psychiatry of Today, and The Psychiatry of the Future. I will limit myself to commenting on the fourth and final chapter (which, in a sense, also encompasses the others).

What should the psychiatry of the future keep in mind? the author asks. His legacy (or manifesto) can be summarized in six points.

One: the use of phenomenological insight. Placing patients' experiences, emotions, and stories at the center of care, bracketing the illness in order to get closer to its essence, which continues to elude cold, biological assessment.

Two: the practice of gentle listening. Receiving patients' suffering, expressed verbally and nonverbally, in silences, words, and facial expressions, with engagement and empathy. There is no therapy outside of therapeutic conversation based on listening.

Three: recognizing the value of words. Being aware of the power of words in relationships of care: words are living creatures, they can hurt or open up to hope. This is why Borgna speaks of "madness" rather than "mental illness" or "schizophrenia," a word that still carries stigma today.

Four: the value of poetry and great novels. Literature allows psychiatry to expand its knowledge of the spirit, helping it to approach the mystery of subjectivities wounded by the pain of anguish and distress.

Five: fragility as a secret dimension of madness. Madness is fragile, not violent: we must debunk the dominant association between madness and violence. It is fragile, and yet it reveals profound realities of the human condition that would otherwise remain hidden.

Six: the community of care and of destiny. A community must be created of those who provide care and those who are cared for, recognizing ourselves in the destiny of the other's fragility, feeling and experiencing their pain and anguish as if they were, at least in part, also our own.

What, then, should be excluded in the psychiatry of the future?

All forms of restraint (physical, chemical), violence (including verbal) against the mind or body, such as electroshock. In a word: the asylum, which, even before being a non-place, is a *forma mentis*.

Eugenio Borgna brought a human face back to madness, reestablishing psychiatry as a humanistic science as well as a natural one. He redeemed kindness and listening: values and categories that go far beyond psychiatry. His books testify to this, proclaiming the scandalous and revolutionary news that "madness is not something extraneous to life, it is a human possibility within each of us, with its shadows and its emotional incandescence. The distance, the separation between psychotic and non-psychotic life is sometimes only quantitative, not qualitative. Sorrow and anguish are human experiences all of us are familiar with."

Introduction
The Threshold

As I set forth on the path of the various forms my life in psychiatry has taken, I would like to point out a few thematic constants. This introduction, which attempts to put into the simplest possible words what the thing called phenomenological psychiatry is, or at least how it can be interpreted—the same phenomenological psychiatry that led to the revolutionary reform law in Italian psychiatry—will be followed by four chapters, along with some final reflections.

Initially, after brief reflection on the meaning of the psychiatric revolution, we will proceed to reconstruct the bases of the psychiatry of the past, their historical connotations and in particular my own experiences at the clinic for nervous and mental disorders at the University of Milan, where psychiatric and neurological instruction were interwoven, and later in a psychiatric hospital, or asylum, as it was called then, in Novara. Those were years when psychiatry was considered—and in essence, this hasn't changed—last among the medical specialties, and psychiatry as practiced in the asylums (the historical and semantic echoes of this term compel me to retain it), the institutionalized treatment of madness, nonetheless inadequate to address the clinical problems and human sources of madness. My pages will tell how in the clinic in Novara, the dignity and freedom of the patients—I was always assigned to the women's section—were never encroached upon, and were always respected. My pages here will speak of how my encounter with madness revealed to me its fragility and weakness, its sensitivity and kindness, its spiritual aching and defenseless resignation before the neglect and indifference of normal people who are, not seldom, the bearers of conscious or unconscious violence. Madness in women particularly carries emotional and psychopathological resonances, as we know, among other things, from the famous descriptions of the madness of Ellen West, Suzanne Urban, and Ilse and Lola Voss, salvaged for the history of psychiatry by the famous Swiss psychologist Ludwig Binswanger, to whom we owe the phenomenological and human reformulation of psychiatry which is, however much forgotten or ignored, a part of the psychiatry of the past.

The investigation that follows is centered on the radical changes that followed the 1978 legal reform that led to the closure of the asylums and the creation of psychiatric hospital services on par with other medical specialties, the opening of assisted living facilities, and the organization of a network of outpatient clinics that allowed patients to be treated, in emergency cases, at their private residence. In the second part of the present work, I examine these unimaginable changes in psychiatric method and technique that followed the revolutionary theoretical and practical insights of Franco Basaglia, who has shown how, in his beautiful words, the impossible can become possible. There are still deficits in the practice of Italian psychiatry, but they can in no way be compared with the intolerable conditions of the Italian asylums, even if not all of them were so bad, such as the women's ward in Novara.

And what of the psychiatry of the future? It must be a psychiatry that that overcomes the precarity of certain treatment models in psychiatric hospital services; that ideally restores momentum to those aspects of the reform law not yet fully carried out; that is bold in its increasing awareness of the importance of words and silence in the structuring of care; that tends, with a Leopardian passion for hope, to an acceptance of the fragility and human dimension of madness, not forgetting Clemens Brentano's lovely definition of it as poetry's less fortunate sister; finally, a psychiatry of listening that, without dispensing with rigorous pharmacotherapy, emphasizes the impor-tance of psychotherapeutic and sociotherapeutic approaches. To conclude this section, I must dwell not on clinical history, but on the lived experience of two patients whose mental state, whose anguish, whose extreme fragility return to the surface, leading one to choose voluntary death twenty years after the appearance of her illness as the final hope against hope.

These pages have attempted to outline what this book aims to be: *not* a psychiatric text such as would risk obscuring the burning flames of that pain that is the soul (which Schelling defines as the inner sky of man, as Lionello

Sozzi writes in his beautiful book) of every human condition of suffering, but the *itinerarium cordis* of a psychiatry on a relentless and impossible search for the mystery of madness.

In an unspeakably beautiful verse by Eugenio Montale, there glimmers an image of acedia that seems mirror the shadows of melancholy and sorrow, fragility and spiritual turmoil, wounded nostalgia and shattered hope, which are the visible and invisible traces of that condition of life which we call, with dreadful frivolity, madness: "Often I've encountered evil: / it was the stream that chokes and roars, / the shriveling of the scorched leaf, the fallen horse."

Let me add here that psychiatry cannot refuse the assistance of poetry in recognizing the fragility and humanity of madness: madness in its mildest forms as well as its most painful.

I. The Revolution in Psychiatry

The first revolution in psychiatry—a revolution not just of knowledge, but of ethics—took place at the beginning of the past century in phenomenology's wake and radically changed the object of psychiatry, which turned away from the brain and its dysfunctions and toward patients' subjectivity, their interiority, their way of being in the world of interpersonal relations. Redefining it as a human science and not simply a natural one was possible thanks to the insight of certain psychiatrists from the previous century who drew on philosophy, and on phenomenology in general, to identify and illuminate psychiatry's human origins. But as the years passed, this cultural revolution failed to take root concretely in psychological practice, which continued to refer to or follow theoretical and practical models of somatological psychology, its reduction to a natural science and to a discipline largely assimilable to neurology. Psychiatry in the asylums, a psychiatry of madness's exclusion and negation of meaning, was entirely an implementation of the theoretical and practical reasoning of somatological psychiatry. In European countries, particularly Italy and France, this conception of psychiatry found its most rigid and often terrifying expressions in the establishment of asylums where people's dignity was daily violated in thrall not only to a hollow psychopathological incivility but also to a theoretical conception that deemed psychic suffering (or *mental illness*, a term that remains as heartbreaking as it is scientifically unsettling) as incurable and essentially untreatable. Only in Italy, only in the revolution brought about by Franco Basaglia and officially established by Law 180 of May 1978, did phenomenology emerge from the closed laboratories of thought and intuition to provoke a radical change in our way of treating psychic suffering, valuing its inalienable dignity and its liberty, which was under siege but not lost.

Phenomenological Themes

The phenomenological themes that emerged were particularly the following: respect for the dignity of suffering; the awareness that madness is part of the human condition; the bracketing (this idea comes from Husserl) of illness which allows us to approach its essence, its deeper nature, and its trembling humanity; the radical importance of introspection and empathy in the comprehension of lived experiences in ourselves and others; and the decisive significance of human interactions in treatment. These theoretical orientations converged in an extraordinary transformation of psychiatry that—heterogony of ends—in Italy, where asylum psychiatry's bequest had been painful and inhuman, came to a rediscovery of ideals that seemed almost utopian, yet instead led to the eventual closure of the asylums.

Phenomenology in psychiatry throughout most of the twentieth century was little more than a fragile if very humane alternative to somatological psychiatry, producing texts of extraordinary psychopathological and human depth that allowed us to recognize not only in neurotic, but also in psychotic experiences, in madness *tout court*, forms of life sealed by pain, but ever anarchic, always endowed with meaning. In this connection, I would like to recall the clinical life histories of Suzanne Urban and Ellen West, who were trapped in the burning bushes of schizophrenia and whose existential vicissitudes are masterfully described by Ludwig Binswanger, as well as the experience of a young schizophrenic, Elena, expertly depicted by Enrico Morselli, my predecessor as chief of the psychiatric hospital in Novara. Still today, we read these clinical histories with amazement, and they lead us to recognize that even in schizophrenia, the sphinx of psychiatry, the human path proceeds in pain and endowed with sense. Phenomenology allows us to outline and analyze these clinical histories with a radicality and profundity that take us into the very heart of madness, revealing its disturbing emotional dimensions in their sensitivity, psychic pain, and humanity.

From the expansive regions of phenomenology I would like to draw out certain of its components that will help show how it can be a path to psychiatric knowledge.

The Phenomenology of Dialogue

There are words that linguists refer to as compound or portmanteau words with multiple semantic horizons, and dialogue ("colloquio") could be considered one of these. Following Hölderlin's famous verse ("Seit ein Gespräch wir sind," meaning that we, people, are conversation) leads to other definitions: exchange, relation, encounter, identification, and so on, thematized in their emotional and rational totality by listening and that attention that Simone Weil described as a form of prayer.

Dialogue, a dialogic way of being, is phenomenology's bequest to the form of psychiatry that seeks to be humane and kind; and I would like to speak now of certain phenomenological models of dialogue. The phenomenological dialogue does not arise in a desert or in a void, but in the here-and-now of time and space. The meaning of words changes to the degree that they come up against the time and space of the other, whose words distance us, bring us closer. And not just that: the desire for solitude (for distance from the world and from others) and the desire for communication (for closeness to the world and to others) are interwoven, and only emotional awareness can tell us when it's time to speak and when it's time to be silent; when to employ the language of words, and when to employ the language of the lived, signifying body. Insofar as he is a living essence, man is capable of entering into conversation with another to bring into the light of language that which disturbs him, as Shakespeare says beautifully in Macbeth: "Give sorrow words; the grief that does not speak whispers the o'er-fraught heart and bids it break."

The work of reciprocal coming-to-consciousness in therapeutic dialogue takes place not in an atmosphere of arid intellectuality; it is linked to the emotions; and in the course of conversation something new always emerges. We are inundated with emotion, and we need to trust the person treating us, with no fear of indifference or apathy as that person hears of the weaknesses that may make us feel ashamed or guilty. The qualities one ought to expect from a psychiatrist are patience, discretion, human warmth, introspection, and empathy, the capacity to create a climate of trust and of comprehensive listening that never dismisses the other's words. These are spiritual inclinations, ways of being that are radically phenomenological at their core, and every therapist and (I believe) every doctor must be aware of them if they intend to enter into a dialogical relationship with their patients. For the extent of technological progress has made us forget the irreplaceable importance of dialogue, the healing word, not only in psychiatry but in medicine as well.

Phenomenology, Again

Nor is phenomenology alien to the way in which psychiatry apprehends the meaning of illness, or lack thereof. Ought we consider illness in its radically pathological nature, or as a phenomenon that characterizes the fragility of the human condition? Our perception of illness decides whether the therapeutic relationship will be shaped by emotional proximity or distance, affinity or disaffinity; and the therapeutic relationship is influenced by the attribution or non-attribution of horizons of meaning to a given symptom; matters that clinical psychiatry of both the past and present have all but ignored.

Phenomenology can only view psychic suffering, and psychotic episodes in particular, in its fragility and longing for human kindness. Thus, something only apparently banal or rhapsodic is necessary so that a patient, whose trust we wish to earn, not be asked questions that would feel like intrusions or violations of their timidity—but we must also consider what meanings the patient assigns to their delusions and hallucinations. These are symptoms that neuroleptic drugs may often reduce to a greater or lesser extent, but their elimination is not always advisable. When patients have adapted to the presence of delusions and hallucinations, their disappearance sometimes causes an unexpected reemergence of anxieties and disturbances that may lead to suicide. I must agree here with the thesis of a Swiss psychiatrist of the past century: better to fight deluded with the entire world than to be alone. Such an assertion is possible only when one has immersed oneself in the inner life of patients, in the search for the meaning that delusions and hallucinations possess.

The Phenomenology of Emotions

Modern thought considers emotions, passions, intuitions to be categories that reveal meaning and fate. Giacomo Leopardi expresses this perspective radically. "But reason is never as effective as passion. Listen to the philosophers. Men should be led to act in accordance with reason as much as, indeed much more than, out of passion; in fact, their actions should be determined solely by reason and duty. Nonsense." And: "Rather than extinguish passion with reason, it would be better to turn reason into passion: to make duty, virtue, heroism, etc., become passions." And finally, "pure, unadulterated reason is a direct source of inevitable and total madness, and is so by its own nature."

How do we recognize and understand the emotions, the passions (which are emotions that persist in time) that live in us and those that live by virtue of ourselves in others? How may we set forth on the paths that lead into the peaks of our interiority? Only if we know how to teach ourselves to grasp something of that which shifts in the deepest parts of our inner selves will we be able to recognize the infinite and not seldom ungraspable cascade of our emotions; and we must not tire of looking into ourselves, of this continuous, at times wearisome, at times distressing search for what we are in the vast regions of our emotions. We know their twists and turns only if we know how to live in solitude within ourselves, and for this reason, I would like to recall the words of Rainer Maria Rilke: "For there is only one solitude, and it is large and not easy to bear." And: "What is needed is only this: solitude, great inner solitude. Going within and meeting no one else for hours — that is what one must learn to attain."

Phenomenology in psychiatry drives us to grasp those meanings that are unseen, beyond every visible threshold, hidden in us, and outside of us, and without an ardent, febrile searching for values and meanings, which come alive within us, psychiatry cannot realize its ends and its destiny, which are to lend a hand, as Manfred Bleuler says, to the person descending into the abysses of madness. Without this quest that brings us together, despite all differences, with the appearances and disappearances, the ghosts and shadows, the pain and suffering of melancholy and anguish, it is impossible to help the ill person or to safeguard our inwardness, which tends to wither and fade away. It is a tool of exhausted technologies that exclude the soul from the discourse of care, that soul that perhaps is hiding in the anxieties of the hearts in those who give treatment, as well as in the hearts of those who receive it. The ways of living our own emotions are mirrored in the ways of being of the body: of the living body, of the signifying body.

The Phenomenology of the Body

Phenomenology is always interested in the body, not the physical body, the body-thing, the body-object, but the living body, my hand which suddenly springs into action and communicates something: my anxiety, my sorrow, my joy, my impatience, my expectation, my hope. But what are we to say of the face, the gazes, the tears, the smiles—of these ways the living body expresses itself that phenomenology, as the passion for difference, has rediscovered and made known in expressions of such radical importance as psychiatric diagnoses? As I progress through the present work, I would like to point to certain aspects of phenomenology, the north star of my book, and I will also draw literary testimony, certain of its emblematic expressions of the living body, and of the face in particular, as in this fragment from the great Hungarian writer Sándor Márai's beautiful novel, *Casanova in Bolzano*, in which Francesca says to Giacomo: "Because we are still only masked figures, my love, and there are many more masks between us, each of which must, one by one, be discarded, before we can finally know each other's true, naked faces." And then: "Don't hurry, there is no rush, no need to grope for the mask you are wearing or to throw it away. It is no accident that we are wearing masks, meeting, as we do, after a long time, when both of us have escaped our prisons to face each other: we needn't hurry to throw away our masks, because we will only find other masks beneath them, masks made of flesh and bone and yet as much a mask as these, made of silk." Finally, with a stunning image that grasps an everyday aspect of the face: "There are so many masks we have to discard before I can get to see and recognize your face." This is the phenomenology that tells us how we are responsible for the faces of others, as in Emmanuel Lévinas's noted formulation, which mirrors our emotions, sometimes against our will.

The Phenomenology of Time

The legacy of phenomenology also concerns the ways patients experience time, not the time of the clock, the time of the hourglass, but the time of the self, lived time, which in melancholy, in its diverse forms of expression, undergoes profound alterations, as we must never forget. Time ceases to evolve, there is no more future, only a present and a past, with the consequent spread of feelings of guilt and the foundering of hope as openness to the future and to change. Lived time is radically modified in mania in which past and future go unlived as one pursues an eternal present that no longer has meaning. These are the modifications of lived time that Eugène Minkowski masterfully analyzes and describes in one of his most important works. What takes place, on the other hand, in schizophrenia, the most enig-matic of psychic maladies? Time crumbles, breaks apart, splinters, and the perception of oneself and the world is profoundly deformed; phenomenology attests to this in ways that ought not be ignored. I will limit myself to these considerations of time, the modified experience of time, which occurs in disturbances that phenomenologically-oriented psychology addresses in its search for a meaning that we should be primed to catch sight of in madness.

The Phenomenology of Space

In the unfolding of psychotic experiences, space, and not only time, is per-ceived as different from the one we all live in, and phenomenology allows us to grasp these differences. It has nothing to do with geographical or geo-metrical space, but with lived space as a source of meaning. Its vertiginous expansion, its flattening, its rigidity, its kinship to the suggestive experience of infinitude, its petrification and liquification, are some of the modes of experiencing or not experiencing space in certain forms of psychotic life. The bodily figures of people and things lose their spatial consistency and give rise to a world (the inner world and the ambient world) in which the deserts, the Tartar steppe, expand. In the silence and in the liquification of space we see an emblematic image of the outer limits of psychic suffering: those of schizophrenia (a term that ought to be abolished, but remains difficult to replace) and its rending loneliness. In such a condition, there are no longer regions of the soul to serve as anchors in this extreme dilation of lived space, marked by the void produced by the dissolution of corporeal boundaries.

Horizons

In the past century, the philosophical movement of phenomenology marked psychiatry as it radically changed its object of research and treatment, no longer the brain and its disfunctions as in the nineteenth century but rather subjectivity, patients' interiority, the boundless world of emotions, and their way of being in the network of social relations. It was Ludwig Binswanger and Karl Jaspers who built the foundations of phenomenological psychiatry, which, among other things, has humanized the modalities of assistance and care in psychiatry. In the final decades of the past century, phenomenological psychiatry was gradually pushed aside by, on the one hand, pharmacological psychiatry, and by the descriptive and atheoretical psychiatry of the *DSM*, the *Diagnostic and Statistical Manual of Mental Disorders* on the other. Phenomenological psychiatry would have disappeared had it not been revitalized by the work of Franco Basaglia, who extracted it from its theoretical foundations and transformed it into psychiatry as revolutionary praxis—yet without abandoning the phenomenological core that expanded its field of meaning.

Over the course of my considerations here, I have gone looking for what of this phenomenology is still alive, and for what a humane and attentive psychiatry can never do without. Phenomenology, which I will refer back to throughout this book, is grounded in the intuitive and emotional knowledge of lived experiences which, in illness and in health, are mirrored liberally in the wonderful works of Eugène Minkowski.

II. The Psychiatry of Yesterday

In this work, I would like to make some considerations concerning my life during the periods in which it encountered the enigmatic and painful figure of psychiatry: the sadness and anxiety, the unspeakable suffering, and the wounded hope that go hand in hand with psychiatric work, and that, beyond other possible connotations, constitute its deepest core, both its grandeur and its precarity.

The image we have of psychiatry today is no longer that of the past that remains distant but close, when it was considered a discipline centered solely on "mental illnesses" that no one even wanted to hear about. For psychological problems, help was sought from neurology, which is still somewhat true today, and only an elite was aware of psychodynamic approaches to treatment. This is the cultural and social low point that marked the psychiatry of yesterday, where those doctors who chose to live and work as psychiatrists found themselves stranded.

The Well of the Past

In my journey back into the past, my search for lost time, I cannot forgot what Thomas Mann wrote in the opening pages of his most complex and imponderable novel—a novel that yields only with difficulty to reading: *Joseph and his Brothers*. "Deep is the well of the past. Should we not call it bottomless? Indeed we should, if—in fact, perhaps only if—the past subjected to our remarks and inquiries is solely that of humanity, of this enigmatic life-form that comprises our own naturally lusty and preternaturally wretched existence and whose mystery is quite understandably the alpha and omega of all our remarks and inquiries, lending urgency and fire to all our speech, insistence to all our questions."

Obviously my own history has nothing to do with the wells of the past evoked by Thomas Mann, and yet how many things are, and continue to be, mysterious and inscrutable in everyone's past; and so I must now look backward, to a past in which I chose psychiatry, a profession full of shadow and light, expectation and hope, vocation and contradiction.

The Milan University Clinic

I had only a vague understanding of psychiatry apart from the supporting role it played in neurology textbooks, this being a fundamental aspect of university coursework in medicine and surgery; I discovered psychiatry later, after I had graduated from the University of Turin and was specializing in neurology at the clinic for nervous and mental illnesses at the University of Milan. A concentration in psychiatry only appeared some years later. Neurology was the branch of medicine least distant from my philosophical and literary inclinations. In the Milan clinic, some of the beds were assigned to people with mental disturbances: not psychotic, but neurotic. The clinic's orientation was thoroughly neurological, and yet it was not lacking in human sensitivity and attention to the psychological problems of the ill. The clinic's directors, Carlo Riquier and later Gildo Gastaldi, and two assistants in particular, Lorenzo Cazzullo and Italo Sanguineti, followed us interns with kindness and passion, and their teachings have formed part of my life: they were my mentors in culture and humanity.

The Asylum of Milan

I would nevertheless not have become familiar with psychiatry, psychiatry proper, had the aforementioned Carlo Lorenzo Cazzullo, who passed on to me the importance of passion and rigor in scientific research, openness to the human and the primary role of ethics in the sciences, not assigned me to study the therapeutic effect of psychotropic drugs, which had been discovered in those crucial years, on the lives of psychotics, in a psychiatric hospital in Milan, then considered one of the most forward-looking of the now-shuttered asylums in the city. It was a shocking image of inhumanity and glacial indifference to the values of dignity and human sensitivity, one that would never be erased. Of course, having been sent by the clinic, I could read the medical records, which in their inconsistency said nothing about the patients' states of mind, and I was able to talk to them, analyzing and describing their emotions, marked by pain, and despair, nostalgia, and loneliness of the soul. Eventually I compiled this research in a monograph focusing on the clinical and therapeutic, but also the psychopathological and phenomenological aspects, of psychic suffering: giving voice to madness, drawing it out in its authenticity and its humanity, which my patients' surrounding conditions couldn't erase. In listening to the patients, staying beside them and never paying any attention to the clock, how much anguish I heard, how much suffering, how much sadness and how much despair, how much loneliness and how much longing for words and gestures that never came, how much kindness of soul in their faces and expressions, dulled and exhausted by pain. The most disturbing thing of all, which even today lingers in my memory, was being called to stand by during electroshock treatments, which at the time was the preferred therapy for depression as well as for schizophrenia (and is still practiced in university hospitals and private clinics, but with anesthesia). In an appallingly large room with who knows how many patients, standing side by side, one after the other, observing the others' convulsive fits, in the cold and futile indifference of the doctors who took turns administering electroshock. To imagine the fragility and the delicacy, the sensitivity and the vulnerability, the frightened resignation and the disorientation of the patients tugged at one's heart, and I asked myself if this was still psychiatry.

The Clinic Again

What was madness, in the eyes of the psychiatrists working in this asylum, but anarchy and senselessness, biological disturbances and isolation impenetrable to environmental influence, so that any and all dialogue, any and all relations were pointless? When my research was at an end, and I had grown aware of the horrors of psychiatry and the human sensibility of madness, I returned to the clinic, and gradually the anguished, desperate images of life in the asylum receded from my wounded memory: images of the patients' bottomless suffering and the glacial indifference of those taking care of them.

At the time, I was still in the field of neurology, the most rigorous and math-ematical of the medical disciplines, writing works, sometimes in conjunction with the Institute of Pathological Anatomy, entirely distant from psychiatry, but that permitted me to acquire the neurobiological education necessary for the often painstaking differential diagnoses between psychological and neurological disturbances. At the same time, I was reading the great works of psychiatry and of psychopathology, which is the soul of psychiatry, in German, along with those very few texts in Italian that were worth perusal and study: those of Ferdinando Barison, Franco Basaglia, Bruno Callieri, Danilo Cargnello, and Enrico Morselli. That's all there was in Italy, apart from the wonderful novels of Mario Tobino, which described in lyrical and inspired words the painful and agonizing aspects of madness as well as the creative and human ones.

My years of study and in the clinic came to a summit of practical expe-rience and theoretical awareness, and in 1962, at thirty-two years old, I was appointed to a teaching position in nervous and mental disturbances at the clinic. I could have chosen the far from easy path of a university career, but you cannot always predict what form your life will take.

The Turn

The painful and bitter experience of the asylum in Milan had brought me into contact with the horrors of psychiatry and the human grandeur of mad-ness (in those years, *Esprit*, the magazine founded by Emmanuel Mounier, devoted a wonderful issue to the splendors and miseries of psychiatry) and so, knowing there was an opening for a clinician in the asylum in Novara, I was tempted to apply. It was a bold challenge, and success was barely possible. Enrico Morselli had been director there since 1935 (and would remain there until 1970); he came to Novara from the university clinic for nervous and mental illness in Milan, following a path that could have been my own. Known across Europe as well as in the United States, Morselli was the author of tremendous, beautifully written works that remain relevant today, highly original books in Italian and French about schizophrenia and mescaline addiction, the relationship between literary-artistic experiences and psychosis, and psychiatry as a human science and not only a natural one. Before the final selection was made, I went to his study in Novara one day, and in an immense room with walls covered in famous paintings, a large dog crouching at his feet, Morselli greeted me, very tall and very thin, smiling, and his passion for hope, his belief in a humane and kind psychiatry, shone in his sometimes fragile words, his eyes, and his way of seeing. One could not help but be fascinated by his culture, his spontaneity, and his timidity, which revealed itself particularly when he had to speak in public, showing the mysterious syntony of his way of being and of writing.

Elena

His best work, of incandescent emotional tension, was published in 1930, and even today, we read it with apprehension. It follows the schizophrenic experience of Elena, a twenty-five-year old Italian pianist who was hospitalized at the University of Milan neuropsychiatric clinic from May 1925 to July 1927. In dissociative states, she expressed herself sometimes in Italian and sometimes in French. Elena's experiences are described in their vital raison d'être and in her sequences of interwoven normal and pathological life. In her French phases, her symptoms increased, causing her to lose all contact with reality, whereas in her Italian phases, they abated, and she adapted better to her environment. The other world of madness reemerged with emblematic semantic resonance in listening to oneiric and arcane, luminous and painful words, pathological and yet not alien to the life that is in each of us. A patient is not a *thing*, not a diseased *organ*, but a person with an inner life, and the anxiety and suffering, uniqueness, and longing for connection that come with it. This is the authentic dimension of existence that includes yet transcends the symptomatologic dimension of schizophrenia when analyzed by Morselli with his remarkable insight and listening skill. His work revives the radical importance of language in psychiatry, and only a language that is elevated and rigorous, metaphorical and even lyrical, can give Elena an image that in another style would have been withered and empty. From this luminous diary reemerges the figure of a patient, her experiences, and her world, in her soul's turmoil and her despair. Enrico Morselli was able to reveal the human meaning of illness in psychiatry, at a time—not limited to the years of Elena's clinical condition—when Italian psychiatry was drawn toward a cold positivistic logic. This was one of its historically unforgettable merits, along with having shown that, in schizophrenia, life continues to attest to its wounded, aching, meaningful grandness. Morselli demonstrated the possibility of care, of care as dialogue, which brings us to the depths of pain and anguish of those who live with schizophrenia, furthermore at a time when antipsychotic drugs didn't yet exist.

Hallucinations

From Morselli's clinical diary, I would like to excerpt certain considerations on patients' hallucinations. "Elena experiences phenomena of hallucinatory disturbance with remarkable lucidity and awareness (also tactile and synesthetic: she sees little spiders and creeping insects); a hole appears in the ceiling, "it's death!"; she feels herself being touched, mysteriously embraced, keeps her eyes closed as if she cannot see. She's highly excitable, the strangest sensations invade her; the slightest noise generates violent reactions; she no longer recognizes her own or my voice, she becomes disoriented in the room. She'll say that "that evening" that was how she felt... and she says she doesn't speak French, she doesn't feel like speaking French... Her state of consciousness doesn't seem altered; she remembers (in occasional moments of respite) everything that happened that day." When Morselli asked her which was the true Elena, she answered that both the one who spoke Italian and the one who spoke French were true. Of course, if this had been typical of Italian psychiatry, if this had been the way Italian psychiatrists—at least some of them—listened to their patients, going over their delusions and hallucinations, their spiritual anguish and pain together, Italian asylums would not have been the non-places that they were.

The Asylum in Novara

And so, a year after taking on the teaching position, I entered the asylum of Novara: as head physician in 1963, and as director in 1970, and I held this position until 1978, when Law 180 mandated the closing of the asylums, at which point I became head physician in psychiatric services of the Ospedale Maggiore in Novara. The women's section of the asylum, where I had carried out my work, was reorganized in 1970 as the second psychiatric hospital in Novara, separate from the men's, with its own independent management.

On a late afternoon in the autumn of 1963, I was walking down the silent, subdued tree-lined roads of the Novara Asylum, immersed in the green lawns and the infinite songs of the lonely sparrows. The immense structure stood outlined mysteriously against the scarlet backdrop of the sky, three floors of barred windows that gave glimpses of the faces of the patients who had been there for so long. The bars were cruel and unmoving, the cracked windows were silent and empty, but then, out of nowhere, the faces and eyes of the patients would light up and would seem to erase that prison of bars and windows. Suddenly it was as if I were entering another world, a world enclosed in pain, silence, and solitude, far from quotidian distractions and banality. Since then, rivers of experience have marked my life, leaving behind burnt ashes, but the emotions I felt in my unsettling entrance into the unknown world of madness have never withered in their uncontaminated turmoil.

When later I walked through the halls and rooms of the asylum, I was struck by the patients' fragility and kindness, their timidity and the sensitivity. I was always employed in the women's wards, where there was nothing of the glacial indifference or the terrifying electroshock treatments that I had seen in the asylum in Milan. The doors were locked, some patients were confined, the long-term inmates lived in conditions very different from those of the short-term ones, but the emotional atmosphere was one of listening and not of violence: nuns and nurses approached the patients with kindness and humanity, and the doctors did as well. Therapy was pharmacological, and electroshock wasn't used.

An Aside

I insist: not all asylums were like the one in Milan, however much people continue to think and say so even today. In the asylum in Novara, even under the directorship of Enrico Morselli, in years when psychic suffering was considered to be of biological origin, and every treatment except shock therapy was deemed useless, there never would have occurred such things as one saw in the asylum of Sant'Antonio Abate in Teramo, where rebellious and free-acting women were hospitalized, as Paolo Mieli recalls in the *Corriere della Sera* of December 12, 2017, in his review of a book by Annacarla Valeriano. He writes, "Almost always, diagnoses of 'strange behavior owing undoubtedly to mental imbalance' (or something of the sort) were sufficient to lock up many of these poor people in publicly funded concentration camps for the mentally ill. By the end of the 1960s, some young people were hospitalized by force for abandoning home and work 'to join the hippies' or because they had gone 'to seedy nightspots for sex.' This situation persisted, more or less, for many years, practically until May 13, 1978, when the so-called Basaglia Law was passed. Incredible." Obviously, one cannot deny observations like these, which are based on the clinical reports of the asylum in Teramo, but one cannot generalize either. In Novara, even before it became part of the Milan University clinic, there was never anything comparable to what is described here, and so it is unfair to describe all psychiatric hospitals as instruments to punish "female behaviors considered transgressive."

It is true that, during the fatal war years, Jewish people with no patho-logical traits whatsoever were interned in the asylum in Novara, but this allowed Morselli to save them from persecution and possibly death, and putting himself in grave personal danger by doing so. I feel compelled to mention this to convey that not all asylums, and certainly not Novara (I have already spoken of Enrico Morselli's kindness, sensitivity, and fragility, which would never have tolerated any form of violence), employed the kinds of internment criteria seen in Teramo: these criteria that were unimaginably insensitive, indiscriminately absurd, pointlessly violent. These are things I must say; I feel it is my duty to this asylum director, who was a great teacher of psychiatry but also of humanity, even if today he is regrettably ignored and forgotten. His essay on Elena, the young schizophrenic he treated is unspeakably beautiful, even aesthetically, and should be read and studied not only by all psychiatrists but also by anyone who wishes to know something about the emotional bases of schizophrenia.

Now I would like to return to my life as part of the asylum, from the moment I stepped through its doors and immersed myself in its dark lakes of pain and anguish, but also of hope.

Sources of Pain

I was assigned patients who were entering the asylum for the first time, as well as those who had returned with acute-onset disturbances, and *not* those who had been hospitalized long-term and were, in the unfortunate expression, "chronic." These last I took on only after 1970, when I became director of the women's asylum, and could, with the help of young psychiatrists who had come from the psychiatric clinic of the University of Milan, now independent of the clinic for nervous and mental disorders, transform the model for attending to and treating all the patients and not only the acute ones.

The clinical reports, ours and those written by Morselli in his time, described not only the patients' behavior, but their life stories, their emotions, their moods, their anxieties and longings, their shattered illusions and broken hopes, and were nothing like the dry and meaningless clinical reports of those asylums that had not a trace of humanity, let alone scientific rigor or culture. In an asylum where psychiatry constituted a sincere attempt to empathize with the sources of pain—the thematic core of madness—it was possible to practice a psychiatry animated by dialogue and by the search for words and gestures centered on the opening of hope as a listening to the infinite.

A Brief Period

And psychiatry in the asylum could be this as well: a secret and (almost) invisible source of humanity and kindness, of listening and of the silence of the heart, of a therapeutic community and perhaps a community of fate, apart from the brief period, darkened by unspeakable violence and negligence by a large number of psychiatrists incapable of immersing themselves in the infinite pain of madness. This madness touched me, its grandeur, its dignity, as well as by the reading of texts by the great psychiatrists of the German and Dutch language who spoke of a psychiatry so distant from that which was practiced in Italian and French asylums. Among others, I would like to recall here: Ludwig Binswanger, Karl Jaspers, Eugène Minkowski, V. E. von Gebsattel, H. C. Rümke, Kurt Schneider, Erwin Straus, and Jakob Wyrsch, who radically changed the clinical and psychopathological physiognomy of psychiatry from a natural science to one that was also human. Following the bright footsteps of these greats of psychiatry, the years from 1963 to 1970 were those of the painful discovery of a madness not disdainful of kindness and fragility. These were the years when I wrote my works on depression, schizophrenia, and mania, the years when I worked hand in hand with psychiatrists and psychologists, social workers and nurses, nuns and teachers, with a common horizon of hope and care, of solidarity and ethics.

Women's Madness

It was possible to devote to every patient the necessary time and attention, to listen in a way that was rich with passion and rigor. True, women's madness lacks the harshness and aggressivity so often to be found in men's, and the nurses possessed the sensitivity and tenderness, the kindness and attentiveness, to keep their patience and their desire to relate to their charges; and I cannot omit the nuns, whose tenderness and innate grace I have never forgotten. In those years I was able to practice a psychiatry, focusing on psychotic experiences, that was full of humanity, without bending to non-therapeutic demands. In those years, I was able to reconstruct the life stories of Angela, Anna, Giuliana, Liliana, Margherita, Maria, Maria Teresa, Paola, Valeria, and many other patients, along with the clinical phenomenology of the disturbances that had brought them to the psychiatric hospital, learning to recognize their tenderness and suffering, their sensitivity and despair. Listening and reliving madness in its painful and human dimension, which my books have attempted to give voice to, salvaging it from oblivion, in the knowledge that words are so fragile as to last no longer than a sigh. These are considerations touched by the nostalgia for a past that could not survive the deserts of the typical Italian asylum, where hope died, kindness died, the therapeutic spirit died; and salvation could only come by their closure.

Margherita's Poetry

Margherita was a young schizophrenic I looked after in the years when we were together at Novara. She would later die of suicide. I would like to recall here not her hallucinatory and delusional symptomatology, but the poetry that poured forth from her heart mauled by the horror of death, but also by the longing for death. These wounded words speak of the sensitivity and richness of her inner life, which illness did not manage to destroy. This is a burning testament to pain and to hopes shattered in the vain search for impossible splinters of light.

> You touch the bottom
> When you turn indifferent
> Even to your own pain.

When you clutch at death
For a bit of posthumous
Affection.

When there's nothing left to listen to,
Nothing to say, nothing to see.

When a mouth speaks
And the sounds are unheard.

When indifference
Snatches you from life
In the bottoms of nothingness.

When the disgust is so strong
That nothing explains it.

When the pain hushes meekly
And crushed by its silence
Becomes a sort of mercy.

When your arms are outstretched
And you know not what to do with them.

When the tears are as if trapped in your eyes.

When that howl of despair
Becomes soundless
And you shout, shout
But no one hears you.

So you go on squandering your loyalty
and wait in time
with humility.

What does this poem tell us?

These are poetic fragments that bring us closer, more than notes in a diary, to the thesis that the inner world of schizophrenia, of certain schizophrenias, has psychological and human characteristics that we should always attempt to plumb and reveal, just as with all authentic and meaningful expressions of existence, according to Enrico Morselli. These are fragments of an inner world that hallucinations and deliria mask, and that must be drawn out through gentle listening and an intense engagement that never crosses into identification. These fragments tell us, among other things, how much anguish and pain tormented this patient's the soul, apart from the hallucinations and delusions that may or may not have been present, and in any case are never the only symptoms of illness.

A rhapsodic and expansive poem like this one invites us to consider every form of schizophrenic life in its epiphany of infinite pain and in its desperate quest for fragments of dialogue that sweeten its solitude, a source of pain in itself. A poem that tells us how in madness, death, death as the ultimate hope, may be a fragile and audacious companion, and this ought to suffice to induce psychiatrists and non-psychiatrists alike not to hurt, and even less to dismiss, the extreme sensitivity and vulnerable fragility of patients, with words spoken and unspoken alike.

(These are things I cannot cease to insist upon as this book unfolds, even less now, in a quick flashback on the dilemmatic power of words. I would like to quote an excerpt from a wonderful book by Ferruccio Cabibbe, a Jungian psychiatrist who worked with us for three years in Novara, even if *de domo mea*: "I reached the university clinic, where I realized that, along with my 'scientific' training, I had adopted the attitude of a young, self-assured doctor who expressed himself in specialist terms but also in slang. And so, when talking with the director, I would say, for example, that a patient was "schizo" or "para." These were terms used commonly at the university clinic to describe schizophrenia and paranoia. And the director, who was normally warm and smiling, observed: 'I'm surprised that a person like yourself would use such degrading language to refer to our patients.' At the famous clinic, I was taught many things, but that was one they forgot." Words are nothing if not living creatures.)

Administration

After 1970, when Enrico Morselli retired, the administration of the women's psychiatric hospital faced me with the problem of the many long-term patients, and there was a need for major changes that only the reform law of 1978 could bring into effect. In my eight years in administration, with the collaboration of the psychiatrists who came from the Milan university clinic, the doors of all the wards were opened, restraints were made illegal, and patients could walk the halls of the asylum. Those wards dedicated to chronic patients were joined with those where the inmates showed ambivalent behaviors, being at times calm and at others agitated, as well as with others whose symptoms were stubborn and resistant to treatment and those who were very old and whose treatment was adequate. Only through changing therapeutic and social strategies would it have been it possible to discharge those patients who, in any case, even in the years when I was director, lived lives respectful of their frailty and their dignity; they were treated from various clinical and care perspectives, even if the place itself was not suited to their needs. A chronic illness is immediately considered a loss, which makes it easy for hope to die in those who are being treated and those responsible for treatment.

When I was director, I was responsible for these patients too, and I entered the wards where they spent their days, some young, some no longer young, overseen by nurses and nuns but without recreational activities, which we later sought to remedy. I can see them now, phantoms that are still real, in their calm resignation and inertia. They would come up to me, some smiling, some crying, hoping for a greeting, a smile, sometimes for a touch, a handshake; or sometimes they were aggressive. The older patients, stiff and sometimes frozen in their gestures and expressions, still had an intermittent light in their eyes; the younger ones longed feverishly to be greeted with kindness and with clemency.

(Ferruccio Cabibbe has also written wonderful pages on the functional and structural changes we effected in the patients' lives, in his book which still today rings out with a subtle Leopardian passion for hope).

The Year of the Reform

How did the way of practicing psychiatry, of imagining psychiatry, change in May of 1978, when the law was passed mandating the closure of the psychiatric hospitals? I knew the work of Franco Basaglia, and the radical reforms he had carried out in Trieste, which led to similar closures there; but I doubted it would be embraced so quickly. Naturally, I was excited. The fifteen years in the asylum, of living alongside madness, fragility, kindness, pain in body and soul, smiles and tears, so many patients, those who entered and those who left, the young and the old, were at an end, and nothing would survive from that community of care and fate. Would we still have the freedom to devote to each patient the time needed for listening and for a mediating dialogue of awareness and comprehension of the thousand different forms of madness, the freedom to make autonomous decisions concerning the concrete ways of carrying out treatment and helping from one day to the next? Would we still be able to let the patients leave the wards, and in the morning, when we went to meet them, would they still be able to ask in silence for the help of a word, a smile, and perhaps a tear: things that, in a general hospital, would have been considered mawkishness, futile nostalgia for time past, or childish daydreams? Could we still have made ours those arcane words of Manfred Bleuler: the stronger lends a hand to the weaker, and this is psychiatry?

I don't know, but in the besieged fortress of the women's asylum, which nonetheless was free within, we engaged in a gentle, human psychiatry, with radical respect for the dignity of suffering and despair. I didn't know the future, I didn't know if the fear that everything would end arose from my incapacity to adjust to reality and my bewilderment amid open-eyed dreams, which didn't allow me to grasp the concrete alienating dimension of asylum psychiatry.

The law passed in May of 1978, and during the summer I chose to join the psychiatric institute of the Ospedale Maggiore della Carità in Novara as head physician. Fifteen years of life and work, many articles published in the best Italian journals, were now coming to a close, in the awareness that the reform of the asylums wouldn't be enough to breathe new life into Italian psychiatry, which was always inclined to ignore the phenomenological and anthropological dimension.

We Are a Dialogue

What did my years at the asylum teach me? What experiences and what knowledge came to me and accompanied me in the years that followed? How did my memories, my past, influence or shape the future of my life in psychiatry? Those years weren't pointless, because they allowed me to learn the deep roots of madness, depression, mania, dissociative disorders as a way of living, which on the female side assume a more painful yet clearer shape, gentler and more creative. And they also allowed me to follow in time the birth and death, the evolution and stagnation, the transformation of the symptoms and ways of being of illness, listening endlessly to patients, accepting their weariness with living and their fragility, their sensitivity and kindness, their infinite suffering and dignity, their desire and nostalgia for a life free of pain and solitude. I couldn't have written my works without those years in the asylum, which taught me, among other things, how important it is in psychiatry and in life to know oneself, to seek out the emotions that accompany our thoughts and actions and are endlessly interwoven with our rational choices.

Changing the nurses' practices, helping them to grasp the fragility and sensitivity of the patients, their anxieties and their spiritual misgivings, changed the patients, in a continuous cycle of lived experience; and this was a consequence of the therapeutic significance of relationships not only in psychiatry, but in everyday social life. We are a dialogue, in the words of Hölderlin I previously invoked, and we are particularly so when the loneliness that arises from suffering and illness takes hold of us. But what would be left of these things, these experiences, these expectations, these hopes, these projects, in a psychiatry reconfigured according to the model of a general hospital with its instructions and norms?

The Magic Mountain

My life in the asylum made of these things an essential part of my way of practicing psychiatry, but what traces did this leave in the years that followed in vertiginous succession? Did I manage to free myself from the bewitched allure of those walls in the heart of the city that isolated me from the world of normal life, as if I found myself living in Thomas Mann's magic mountain? One of the great German psychiatrists of the second half of the nineteenth century inclined to draw every possible analogy between psychiatry and philosophy, said that normal life, consumed by conflicts and selfishness, made him wish constantly to return to the asylum, where he found kind and sensitive people, yearning to be helped and listened to, desirous of a handshake and a smile, a tear and a gesture of human solidarity. I would not have taken things so far, but I couldn't shake a nostalgia not unlike such sentiments. An asylum, a strange and perhaps unique one, at least in Italy, with all the limitations of the exclusion of the regular flow of life, became, over time, a community of care and sometimes even a community of fate that brought together doctors and non-doctors, nuns and nurses, with patients, those who came and left, those we had to commit for a greater or lesser length of time.

It was outside of the world, or better still, it was another world, the world of pain and sorrow, of the infinite metamorphoses of sorrow and anguish, wounded nostalgia and resignation, wounded hope and despair. But it was a world where each of us carried on in different ways, from day to day, in fragile and sometimes impossible dialogue with the patients: never restrained, and always respected in their extreme weakness and their anguish, in their unbearable loneliness and their dreams. Obviously, our form of psychiatry did not exclude pharmacological interventions, but the prevailing atmosphere was psychotherapeutic and sociotherapeutic, and moreover, simply human, as these pages of mine will seek to show in the wake of my memories.

Nietzsche

In this reconstruction of the years I spent in the asylum, I am struck to remember how much freedom there was to devote time to each patient: time, clock time, not dictated by economic calculations, but rather carved out from lived time, the time each patient needed, an hour, two hours. In our strange asylum, as in the magic mountain, time, inner time, lived time, had its own way of proceeding, of passing, slow and rich in emotional resonances, and in the evening, thinking over all that had happened that day, the sensation was one not of having wasted time in listening, but of heeding the prayer that Nietzsche claimed to say every morning that he might be of help to someone.

As regard these things (which are easy to deem rhapsodic or idle), I would like to say that in certain ways, psychiatry is quite different from other medical disciplines: for example, in the stress placed on the importance of sensitivity and emotionality, gentleness and mildness, introspection and empathy in the training for this specialty, which matter perhaps more than abstract intelligence, geometry, or mathematics. In psychiatry, the reasons of the heart are no less important than calculating reason, and in it there are conditions so painful and so mortifying that at times the community of care necessarily becomes a community of fate. There is nothing to give a mother inconsolable at the unnatural death of a child but a compassionate ear if she is to bring to light her anguish and her sense of loss, in a dialogue sealed with a silence that can attest to human closeness. That is all I knew how to do when this happened, and naturally I didn't measure the time of such an encounter: but what a psychiatrist gives is nothing compared with what he receives with astonishment in his heart. This last thing one can only speak of with fear and trembling, leaving the final response to silence.

Inner Life

In the practice of psychiatry, it is impossible not to integrate general medical knowledge into the awareness brought forth by inner consciousness: the consciousness of oneself, but also of the emotions and interiority, expectations and hopes, our own and those belonging to the people seeking help from us, a help that is never just medicine, but is also words and silences that open the heart to trust and hope. I am not praising psychology as it was practiced in the asylums in Italy, where for historical and cultural reasons it sank to repulsive levels of inhumanity; I am rather concluding the story of *my* experience in the asylum, which brought me closer to an understanding of the ways of being of madness, psychotic, depressive, and manic experiences, and schizophrenia. I would like to repeat that this was not a comprehension oriented toward the abstract awareness of illness, but rather toward the awareness of the inner life of the patients and their inner experiences, emotions, and lives, in an attempt to retrieve them from oblivion and make known their humanity and their emotional latitudes. The beautiful and painful self-descriptions of the patients attested to in their clinical files have shone a rational light on life experiences which, left unexpressed, would have shattered their hearts, as the plangent words of Macbeth say and as our clinical experiences teach us.

In my years in the asylum, I was also able to definitively confirm the role played by the family and social context *not* in the causation of unipolar and bipolar depression, mania, and schizophrenia, but in facilitating their emergence and determining their evolution, stopping or prolonging them in time. And another thing: what shocking emotion was reborn each time in witnessing the healing of a clinical depression as announced by a smile, by a fragile smile, which suddenly restored the light apparently lost to a face, a face clouded over by pain. And so it must be understood then that my nostalgia is not for *the* asylum, a source of indifference and endless violence, but for *an* asylum incomparable to any other, in which madness seemed at times to vaguely mirror the gentle madness of Maurice Blanchot. There is no phenomenological psychiatry that need not take inspiration from great poetry and fiction, which help it to approach the mystery of subjectivities wounded or wracked by pain and anguish, by sadness and the turmoil of the soul; and my years in the asylum enabled me to grasp the thematic directions of this psychiatry and its horizons of meaning.

The Fragile Reasons of the Heart

Reason brought me inevitably to deem it necessary to close the asylums, which had fallen in Italy to levels of unconscionable inhumanity, but my heart, the fragile reasons of the heart, made me think nostalgically of the lost world of madness that the disappearance of my own asylum, an asylum never consumed by violence and indifference, sparked in my soul, which for fifteen years had dwelled among existences wounded by loneliness and pain and nevertheless open to hope—the passion of the possible (as in the Kierkegaardian definition)—such were my patients, the acute ones and the no-longer-acute ones, and they cannot be erased from a memory captured by those years that were also years of social upheaval. Of course, we should never generalize: in the treatment and assistance of long-term psychiatric patients, reform would have been necessary even in a benign asylum like our own. But is it possible to say the same thing as regards internment for acute psychiatric disturbances? These are subjects examined in the chapters of this book devoted to the psychiatry of yesterday, today, and tomorrow.

Shadows

I would not like now to speak of experiences, of psychiatry in the closed world of the women's asylum in Novara, but rather of the problems I encountered from the time when Law 180 was passed—a law which made room for the best possible psychiatry but certain aspects of which have yet to be implemented even today. Psychiatry, emerging from the besieged citadels of the asylums, entered the ordinary hospitals, and after its extraordinary territorial redeployment, now forms part of the national health service, with the creation of outpatient clinics and centers outside the hospital, becoming more humane and assimilating to other medical disciplines. This has been the most staggering and almost unimaginable revolution in its formulation and its enactment, and it changed everything about Italian psychiatry: such a model has yet to appear in many other countries inside and outside of Europe. We cannot help but be amazed by all that Basaglia managed to accomplish in an incredibly short time, in ways that have never lost their social, human, hermeneutic, and therapeutic significance. But there are painful shadows nonetheless, and I would like to turn to them now.

III. The Psychiatry of Today

In psychiatric hospital services, it has become painfully clear that residential conditions do not always respect patients' human rights. There are psychiatric hospital services even in big cities with locked doors, barred windows, and other hair-raising confinement measures. Basaglia would not have wanted ordinary hospitals to integrate psychiatric services: he feared they would turn into places of separation and exclusion, of violence and containment, where not even asylum norms were respected, and where patients were deprived of their freedom, their dignity, their autonomy, and their hope. General medical facilities were supposed to offer beds, without structure, for those in need of inpatient care. But it didn't turn out that way. It would make no sense to criticize a law that has radically changed and humanized Italian psychiatry, and so I will not do so, but I must observe that its methods are not yet worthy of a psychiatry that is both a social science and a science of intersubjectivity: based on dialogue and listening, on understanding and empathy with the pain and despair of patients.

I write these things so that—or so I would like to believe—young psychiatrists will be aware of the immanent dangers in practicing a psychology at times alien to the inspiration of the reform law, and will know how to courageously challenge those painful upheavals that mar its intentions; they should take particular notice of restraints and the ways they injure and mangle patients' dignity.

Restraint

Restraint is an agonizing problem in psychiatry, in hospital psychiatric services, and in rest homes. It is little talked about; indeed, it is not talked about at all despite its profound and burning ethical dimensions. There are various kinds of restraints, and they can be divided into psychological restraints— employed, among other things, in workplaces; architectural constraints, of which prisons are paradigmatic; pharmaceutical restraints—hard to recognize, but so widespread in psychiatry as to overstep any ethical framework; and physical or mechanical restraints, which are the cruelest and most common, the most painful and the most distressing, and objectively, according to a report by Marco Borghi, Emeritus Professor of law at the University of Fribourg, a form of torture and a flagrant violation of basic human rights. There are distinct levels of physical restraint: it is not my intention to list their disturbing variety, but only to hint at the difficulty of renouncing restraints as a comfortable and apparently safe mode of treatment and of substituting them with human presence: attention and patience, listening and gentleness, a look that tells someone they belong there—in short, love: these are ways of being and acting that can only emerge from the silence of the heart.

How can one fail to see that restraint, a technique radically unacceptable in therapeutic terms, eliminates any possibility of care, adding further suffering to lives already shattered by pain and despair, anguish and sorrow, psychotic dissociation and manic ruin? We must confront this problem if we want to understand how unspeakably they infringe upon human dignity in psychiatry, in the knowledge that there are residents of hospitals and rest homes who are treated and cured without any damage being done to their dignity and their freedom; and that there are others where this doesn't occur, and there is no choice but to turn, when the cries for help become too loud, to the various forms of restraint.

These are things that should lead us to reflect deeply on the abysses of despair that open up when restraint descends like a guillotine on the wounded sensibility and anguish, the longing for life and death, of sick people who are treated as objects, as alter egos deprived of dignity and freedom. One cannot speak of psychiatry as a noble and complex discipline that deals with the depths of suffering and sorrow, of expectations and wounded hopes, if one looks away from its shadows and the harrowing problems brought to the fore by such painful situations as the ways and places in which psychiatry operates in a hospital setting, and what must be done with dissonant behaviors like those that lead to restraint. These are especially salient in the urgent question of aggression, which I would like to reflect upon now.

Aggression

Aggression is a complex, stratified issue that cannot be understood fully in its types of emergence and evolution without taking into consideration its relational basis. Psychotic aggressiveness is the clinical event that most frequently leads to restraining psychiatric patients, and not infrequently in rest homes, where old people are restrained, even only when agitated or complaining. But whether in aggression among psychiatric patients or agitation among the elderly, use of restraint is to some degree motivated by our incapacity to enter into relation with another's way of being and behaving; and so our common ethical task must be directed toward a knowledge of ourselves and a re-cognition of our responsibility for this aggression and agitation. We are tempted to consider restraint as a simple technical safety measure which we apply, or allow to be applied, only in exceptional cases. But this is not the case, and if it were, every instance of restraint, even if only temporary, remains the cause of indelible wounds to the dignity and human rights of persons, and in particular, to those of the fragile and defenseless.

In aggression, relations are of fundamental importance: the willingness to empathize with the emotional life of patients, their expectations, in order to grasp the ideal words and behaviors that will soften their conflictiveness. Much aggression arises from failed relationships with patients, because one is prisoner to routine and indifference, or inwardly empty, or incapable of merciful listening. True relations are those that allow us to enter the inner world of the other, protecting them from basic and banal wounds, which in the painful world of rest homes in particular come among other things from the ways the guests are addressed, without respect, without attention to their hopes, dreams, and longings. The inner vocation to help and heal matters, and it would be better if there were nursing homes and psychiatric hospitals where it was said: "We never restrain, we always embrace." Ethics demands it: but is this utopia or demagoguery? It was possible for Basaglia, and where I worked, in Milan and in Novara, restraints were never used.

Gentle Psychiatry

Psychiatry is an impossible discipline, one that betrays its human reason for being unless we hold such ideal goals as kindness and sensitivity, intuition and grace, imagination and vision, solidarity and hope. These are the principles for helping and healing people fragile and insecure, anguished and desperate, forgotten and marginalized, saddled with cruel and stubborn prejudices, who are deemed insignificant beings and, as history demonstrates, unworthy of living. If we lack these principles, then even the most sophisticated knowledge of pharmaceutical mechanisms of action and the four-hundred-plus diagnoses of the *DSM* will never make us capable of establishing personal relationships with people wounded by pathological anguish and sorrow, by mania and psychotic dissociation, by schizophrenia, which requires listening and dialogue as much as it requires psychopharmaceuticals. Of course, if Basaglia had considered psychiatry to be a biological science rather than a human and social one, he would never have arrived at that revolution that led to the closure of the asylums, which, as I've said, occurred only in Italy, albeit with still unresolved issues, particularly those of psychiatric hospital services with their cold atmosphere of pharmacology, rather than psychotherapy and sociotherapy, and their use of restraint, not only in the pharmacological sense, but still in the cruel physical sense, the unacceptable violence of which I have tried to illustrate.

These faults in method and praxis in such a culturally advanced psychiatry as we have in Italy must be considered alongside the rigidly biological and pharmacological orientation of university psychiatry, which is, in almost all cases, radically alien to the psychopathological, phenomenological, social, and human inspirations of the reform law of 1978. At any rate, I hope that the psychiatry of the future, especially in Italy, is able to rediscover in its theoretical reflections and its concrete forms of action the idealist impulse that led to the reform law, and a passion for hope for every form of psychic suffering, seen from the perspective of its dignity and humanity— its yearning for listening and dialogue.

It must also be said that we are faced with a public opinion increasingly distant from the subject of psychic suffering and incapable of grasping its dialogical and social dimensions, as well as growing neglect from the politicians who had sung the praises of Basaglia's work, grasping its radical ethical foundations and appropriating them for themselves. These are things that should be mentioned in schools, perhaps starting at the elementary level, introducing the nature of psychic suffering and its signs, the fragility and the sensitivity, the wounds of the soul and the human richness that are part of it, and which all of us may face, independently of our age, culture, or social standing—pointing out the importance of gentleness and kindness, smiles and tears, embracing fragility and weakness, expectations and hopes. If this were to happen, the destructive force of prejudices that identify psychic suffering with violence would weaken, as would the fear of confrontation with ways of being and of living in the limitless domains of psychic suffering, of madness, which is interwoven with wounded humanity.

Resonances

These are a few fragmentary reflections on the psychiatry of today, its lights and its shadows, its openings and its closures, its prospects and its faults, its ideals and its failures, but also its horizons of meaning that struggle to live, or to remain alive at all. There is none but fragile knowledge of madness, the genesis of madness, its causes, which are necessarily multiple, vital-historical, psychological, biological, and social; and yet, in this problematic knowledge there is one thing that is undeniable, and it is this: madness, the psychic suffering that nourishes it, is a human experience that forms a part of life, of the life that is within each of us, and must be understood in its deepest nature. The biological foundations can be treated with pharmaceuticals, but also with dialogue, the human encounter between carer and cared-for, self-awareness, emotions that are tested in diverse lived situations, and the readiness to empathize with the feelings of others, to grasp their significance as hidden in the words they use as well as in their body language, expressions and gestures, silences and dreams.

If we condemn psychiatry to be a natural science or a science of behavior, we will never grasp its essence or mystery; and yet, in the specialized schools of psychiatry, as I recalled earlier, there is no research on or assessment of the presence or absence of emotional and cultural readiness or the openness to enter into relation with others, the ability to listen to the low and suppressed voices of pain and silence, to hear the yearning for a friendly gaze, for hope. These are inclinations, qualities, that sometimes, or not seldom, I observed in nuns and in nurses, but not in psychiatrists, who were dominated by their interest in technique.

Mine has always been, and continues to be, a psychiatry based on kindness, an important touchstone in all my work, and listening: a *vox clamans* in the desert, even if this seems to me to be the lifeblood of any psychiatric practice that attempts to grasp not only the diversity but also the ultimate *humanity* of psychic suffering, which still today is approached with diffidence and negligence, indifference and apathy, even with cruelty, with eyes closed to the pain and despair that abide within it.

A Different Psychiatry

It's easy to find oneself trapped in an empty psychiatry of idealistic goals of growth and spiritual maturity and consumed by the application of the endless diagnoses of the *DSM* and the simple administration of psychopharmaceuticals that excludes psychotherapy and sociotherapy. It's impossible for me to conclude this long journey over the paths of today's psychiatry without reflecting, however briefly, on the essential structures of the atheoretical psychiatry of the *DSM*. The various editions, but especially the last one, are indivisible from the exponential growth in diagnoses of psychiatric disturbances.

Allan Frances, head of the task force that compiled the fourth edition of the *DSM*, has written, in a book intended to be a searing response to the fifth, that new, pointless, and dangerous pathologies have been invented without any scientific proof of their clinical reality, leading to a growing demand for psychopharmaceuticals. The epistemological bases of the *DSM* demand that everyone see the same symptoms with the same eyes: symptoms that are found in identical forms all over the world; but sorrow, anguish, guilt, delirium, hallucinations, and suicide are life experiences that shift in diverse psychological and cultural contexts and can only be analyzed in their psychopathological dimensions by starting with the interiority and subjectivity of their sufferer, and not with external behavioral models.

The triumphal embrace of the *DSM*, of its epistemological paradigms, arose, as Allen Frances writes, from its adaptability to the cultural tendencies predominant today: excluding the subjectivity of the choices we make, proposing life models conducive to automatic processes, arriving quickly at predetermined solutions without wasting time searching for the hidden meanings in human realities. There are sufferings that seem pointless to our eyes, but that are full of meaning for those who experience them; and there are hidden sufferings that tear at the soul but that we overlook, distracted by a thousand other superficial matters. I do not know how one can do without research in psychiatry, without intuitive knowledge of the subjectivity, the interiority, of those people who suffer, and are desperately asking for help.

I would like to cite the conclusion of Allen Frances's book on the bitter subject of diagnostic inflation, even diagnostic hyperinflation. "Do we have a realistic chance to reverse diagnostic inflation, or is the die already cast in favor of a never-ending parade of false epidemics? My rational self tells me that diagnostic inflation will win and that saving normal will lose. We opponents to inflation are too few, weak, unfunded, disorganized, and face odds that are impossibly imposing. But then I am reminded of the discouraged army in Henry V—'we few, we happy few, we band of brothers'—who were outmanned six to one but took heart and decisively won the battle of Agincourt." And he concludes, "My two goals—'saving normal' and 'saving psychiatry'—are really one and the same. We can 'save normal' only by 'saving psychiatry,' and we can save psychiatry only by containing it within its proper boundaries. The legacy of Hippocrates rings as true today as it did 2,500 years ago—be modest, know your limitations, and first do no harm. Normal is very much worth saving. And so is psychiatry."

These are words we should never forget, and that measure the radical depth that separates the descriptive psychiatry dominant today from kind psychiatry, phenomenological psychiatry, the psychiatry that is possible to practice in Italy.

People Aren't Objects

At this point, I must quote some of Basaglia's radical remarks on the cognitive paradigms of psychiatry. "This means that, for the psychiatrist, the alternative oscillates between an ideological interpretation of the disease (with the construct of an exact diagnosis obtained through the pigeonholing of the different symptoms into a preconstituted syndromic scheme) and an approach to the mentally ill person in a dimension in which the classification of the disease can or cannot be significant"; and again with striking clarity: "In the first case, once again, we would be accepting an essentially clerical role of the indexing and sorting of files; in the second, we psychiatrists would be seeking out a role we've never had and that would place us—to the degree possible—on the same level as the patient in a space where the category of illness is put aside." These methodological considerations enabled Basaglia to restore freedom and autonomy to psychiatry, and to promote the abolition of asylum psychiatry, in flagrant opposition to the positivist ideology of psychiatry that the various editions of the *DSM* demonstrate.

In addition to the above considerations, I would now like to cite others that demonstrate the ethical and human roots of Basaglia's psychiatry. "Men are not objects that can be arranged in any which order. That is, we must see clearly that man is a social animal, a person, an individual, and a subject." More sharply, and with greater probity, he continues: "Taking things to the point of absurdity, I could feed every person in the world, offer them all a home, create conditions that would satisfy all their material needs, and still, I wouldn't be able to resolve the pain that oppresses them or the distress of their relations with others. This existential angst forms a part of man, it is a reality, and the relationship between the social order and the existential dimension represents the contradiction and opposition of our life. Neither politics nor good will can offer a prescription to resolve such a contradiction."

Legislation of extraordinary human openness such as Law 180, which is inseparable from the thinking and writings of Franco Basaglia (the quoted fragments are a splendid illustration of his unstinting depth and originality), gave rise to a psychology salvaged from biological reductionism and the dry derivation and classification of mental disturbances that the *DSM* has spread across the entire world, and fired by the sparks of human engagement with the fate of psychic suffering and the values of vulnerable humanity it contains.

This concludes the part of this book devoted to the phenomenology of contemporary psychiatry with its extreme highs and lows which nonetheless do not diminish its importance.

Contemporary Psychiatry: The Beginning

In Italy, contemporary psychiatry begins on May 13, 1978, with the reform law coming on the heels of Franco Basaglia's extraordinary work which led to the closure of the asylums. Some months afterward, in October of 1978, I left my post as director of the women's asylum in Novara, becoming head physician at the Ospedale Maggiore della Carità in Novara with, I recall, temporary responsibility for regional psychiatric services, and I remained there until 2002.

The way I practiced psychiatry changed radically: no longer was I in a women's hospital of two hundred beds, but in a ward of fifteen men's and women's beds in spaces so cramped that they barely allowed the patients any freedom of movement whatsoever. A hallway, rooms, normally with two beds, hardly enough for the healing of patients who required long stays. Even now, forty years after the opening of that ward, the spaces have remained the same. In the twenty-four years I served as head physician, the doors of the ward remained open, restraints weren't used, but the medical directors refused to allow the patients to go down to the hospital gardens alone or even escorted.

As director of a psychiatric hospital, I had to answer to the judicial authorities as concerned the legal aspects of hospitalization, but I was completely free in my clinical and therapeutic decision-making and in how much time I devoted to my individual patients, who were allowed to walk in the asylum's immense gardens or visit the city with a chaperone: these things were of no small therapeutic importance. As the head physician of a psychiatric hospital, I had some autonomy in clinical and therapeutic questions but not with regard to the social aspects of the programming, even when this consisted of nothing more than taking patients for a walk in the garden. Maybe this was acceptable from a medical perspective, but it wasn't in the view of a psychiatry conscious of the importance of human relations and their social context to treatment that pharmaceuticals cannot entirely supply, and are at times not even necessary.

The Social Image

The change in the social image, nominally of least importance, was in its own way radical. Running a psychiatric hospital had a societal resonance which, whether for its autonomy and power, the social image it carried, or its vaguely elitist connotation, was despite their differences, not so distant from running a university clinic. Alberto Giannelli, a psychiatrist with whom I began my career at the university clinic in Milan, and with whom I have long been bound by shared ideals and kindred conceptions of a humane and sensitive psychiatry, and author, moreover, of striking works of a broad cultural sensibility, before the age of forty was offered a position as the director of clinical psychiatry at the University of Sassari, which would also allow him to later return to Milan. Nonetheless, he didn't accept the post, choosing instead to take over the leadership of the psychiatric hospital in Bergamo. This was a loss Italian psychiatry would never recover from, as he was the ideal person to bring about radical change, but also a sign of the enduring importance of the administration of asylums in their final years: following what Basaglia had accomplished in Trieste, all of us hoped, in different ways, to be able to do the same things in our asylums. One became an asylum director sometimes via the university clinics—this is how it was in Gorizia, Bergamo, and Novara, but this was no longer the case after the 1978 reform, which increased the number of head psychiatric physicians in hospitals. Those called psychiatrists and trained in specialist programs which are oriented toward teaching pharmacological psychiatry and based on the study of the *DSM*.

In Italy there are no longer lectureships that, if nothing else, as practiced in Germany and Switzerland, required writing anything about psychiatry, a discipline in which one can live and die without ever learning anything new apart from the latest pharmaceuticals that come onto the market, which are often no better than their still therapeutically effective predecessors. And nowadays, general practitioners are free to describe endless anti-anxiety medications and antidepressants.

Medical Directors

In moving psychiatry's therapeutic setting to the contemporary hospital ward, how did relationships with administrations, medical directors, and head physicians in other medical disciplines change? How did relationships among patients change, how did their emotional resonances change in an environment so different from the asylum?

Nothing was as it had been in the asylum: the medical directors, who in Novara changed over the course of the years (there was one of great human and cultural sensitivity who was different, but she didn't last long) viewed psychiatry, as did the majority of the other head physicians, as an irrelevant, anarchic discipline that had little to do with medicine or science, that didn't benefit the hospital, and that only created conflict. The medical directors didn't care about the scarcity of non-therapeutic spaces or what this meant for problematic and complex disturbances such as psychiatry deals with, which require access to open spaces where dialogue can take place.

The years went on and on and the therapeutic spaces didn't change, and the protests against our way of doing psychiatry continued. The differences in the configuration and implementation of asylum psychiatry and hospital psychiatry were radical, among other things because the learning of a health administrator is radically alien to the understanding of the complex problems of psychiatry. Nor was any collaboration with other hospital disciplines possible, as virtually all of them saw psychiatry as fundamentally irrelevant to the practice of medicine.

Now, how could I not have felt that sharp nostalgia for the asylum years I spoke of in the first part of this book, for the freedom and scientific rigor with which we were able to treat our patients, respecting their sensitivities and dignity, their need for dialogue, listening to their expectations and hopes?

(Goodbye, time, goodbye, clock time, goodbye, lived time devoted to listening to patients endlessly, goodbye to the therapeutic community that brought together the asylum, doctors, nurses, social workers, and nuns, so long to the assemblies that united patients and volunteers, young and old, in discussion, goodbye to the walks with patients along the asylum paths—goodbye to a psychiatry that taught us to view madness as an experience that is part of life.)

The Method of Practicing Psychiatry

Now I would like to consider how our way of relating to psychiatric patients at the Ospedale Maggiore in Novara changed. The fragility and the vulnerability of madness, the suffering in its deepest background, were better treated in the humble and forgotten but nonetheless bright and spacious rooms of the old asylum. The reform law closed asylums that had neither therapeutic nor human value, and in those cases, any other treatment would have been better. This is obviously not the first time in the history of ideas that the elimination of one evil, in this case of the asylums, required the sacrifice of a good, of that parcel of humanity that still survived in certain asylums. Basaglia died at the age of fifty-six in 1980, two years after the reform law was passed, and he could not see firsthand, though he predicted it, that hospital psychiatric services would not shed all traces of asylum psychiatry.

But as I've said, in Novara, these traces weren't there: we used no restraints, had no bars on our windows, no locked or barred doors; there was rather an openness to dialogue, to listening, to welcoming and understanding our patients, with whom we created a community of care, however fragile. This was possible, despite the poverty of our facilities, only thanks to a common passion for and a common participation in the mental and physical pain of our patients, their anguish and their sorrow, their despair, which brought together psychiatrists and nurses from the men's and women's asylum under the coordination of a remarkable head nurse from the hospital, Claudia Mantovan, who was gifted with kindness and extraordinary receptivity. The stays were short there, the beds were few, and patients were rapidly discharged, and I yearned for the long conversations that the old asylum had allowed me to have with our patients.

Major depressives could be treated adequately in their acute phase, but things changed when, as sometimes happened, the evolution slowed, above all in the elderly, who were more resistant to the therapeutic effects of antidepressants that were normally well suited to complete clinical resolution. These obstacles and clinical dilemmas nevertheless didn't compel us to infringe upon fundamental ethical and human values. Bipolar disorder brought greater challenges, though. This is a clinical condition in which sadness alternates with pathological arousal and euphoria, which are associated with aggression; such cases require medication, but also need large spaces in which patients can move at ease. Still thornier is the treatment of schizophrenia, the most enigmatic and complex of the psychopathological conditions, and one that requires acceptance and solitude to stem the painful tides of anguish and psychic dissociation. I have examined and analyzed these subjects in many of my works, and wish now only to indicate their essential thematic outlines.

A Few Reflections

The closure of the asylums continues to be an event of historical importance that reminds us of the way psychiatric patients were freed from their chains by Philippe Pinel in Paris on the cusp of the nineteenth century. But this, together with the growing importance of psychiatry in the understanding and treatment of numerous and complex physical maladies, has not sufficed for administrators and medical directors to take an interest in psychiatry and the psychological and social atmospheres and places that psychiatry requires. Financial investment has gone to the major medical, surgical, radiological, and laboratory disciplines and not to the psychologically necessary improvement of living conditions for patients in psychiatric hospitals. Hospital psychiatry in practice awakens no real interest. My ahistorical and archaic-seeming nostalgia for psychiatry as practiced in an asylum such as ours, I repeat, is not such that I cannot say that in Italy, only the closure of the asylums made it possible to imagine and implement a psychiatry adapted to the sensitivity and fragility, the gentleness and vulnerability of madness.

Territorial Psychiatry

If hospital psychiatric services today give rise to the reservations I have outlined as regards the care of patients with acute mental disorders, I cannot fail to reiterate the extraordinary importance of Law 180 in the design and articulation of regional services, which make it possible to follow patients who do not require or no longer require hospital stays on an outpatient basis, in clinics, residential communities, or even at home.

In Novara, regional psychiatry is radically distinct from hospital psychiatry, with outpatient clinics and two residences, each with twenty beds, carrying out its pharmacotherapeutic and psychotherapeutic functions in conditions of acute psychic suffering, and sociotherapeutic functions in conditions that are no longer acute, in the former, now properly renovated, men's ward of the asylum. Community and outpatient clinic are intertwined in a discourse of care that is as gentle and humane as ever, in no way comparable to what I saw in some of the hospital psychiatric wings I have written about. There are open spaces for daily meetings, pleasant entertainments, and socialization, which remove all traces of what these communities were in the past. The beautiful gardens are shared by the psychiatric, forensic, and administrative sections of Novara's local health authority, and the patients in the community crowd them every day. The Novara asylum, unlike almost all others, was not far from the city, but close to its center, and this alone softened its image, making it something like an immense Kafkaesque castle echoing with pain and with hopes that were shattered, but not destroyed.

(The new hospital, which was supposed to replace the one where I spent so many years of my life, is far from the city, in a silent, deserted landscape, and of course, the reform law made it impossible to use it as a treatment site. A hospital like a citadel with its church and its many wings, intended to house who knows how many patients. I was the only one to protest its construction, in vain, and today students and teachers have revived it from the ashes as a school.)

Dissonances

Not all public psychiatry is carried out according to the care and treatment models or ideals of the reform that, in Trieste as well as in Novara, local health authorities are supposed to apply; but one of the incomparable historic merits of the law is its association with the closure of the asylums and the inauguration of hospital psychiatric services with a national model whose care strategy encompasses not only individuals who are unwell, but also families that require assistance and should not be left to fend for themselves. No longer is there a single asylum located far from home; now there are multiple hospitals, outpatient clinics, and residential facilities convenient to reach from one's place of residence. Of course, I contend throughout this work that psychiatry of this kind cannot be carried out other than in the spirit of the great ethical revolution imagined by Basaglia, based on what I will once more call the Leopardian passion for hope, by which psychiatry is experienced as a vocation: an old, wishful, even utopian word, yet one that is essential to understanding limitless forms of suffering the psyche can present. And today this vocation faces a relentless flood of prejudice that makes mountains out of molehills: simply going through a brief period of depression, or being admitted to a psychiatric facility with a depressive diagnosis and released in a matter of days, and a person will be considered mentally ill, in the best of cases, or in the worst, a dangerously mentally ill person who must be avoided: sequestered and isolated. There is no point in insisting that the illness of depression, which many recover from today, can be adequately treated with antidepressants, and that this is different from depression as a mood, which we might just as well call melancholy, sadness, malaise (the German word *Stimmung* here captures a fragile musicality) that isn't pathological but a part of life that and makes us more compassionate and accepting of suffering.

What would Leopardi's poetry, with its inexpressible interweaving of grace, the endless awe it arouses in the heart, be without melancholy, sweet melancholy, but bitter melancholy, too—the melancholy that accompanied him his entire life?

The Impossible Becomes Possible

One of Franco Basaglia's Brazilian lectures seems to me to capture the radical essence of his thought: "The important thing is that we have shown that the impossible can become possible. Ten, fifteen, twenty years back, it was impossible to imagine the asylum could be destroyed. On the other hand, it may yet happen that the asylums will be closed again, even more so than before, I don't know! At any rate, we showed that it is possible to treat madness differently, and this finding is of fundamental importance. I don't believe that an action such as ours is tantamount to definitive victory. But the important thing is something else: knowing what can be done. And I have said a thousand times: we, in our weakness, we as a minority, cannot win. It is always power that wins. At the most, we can persuade. Once when we persuade, we win: we inaugurate a transformative situation from which it is difficult to step back."

These drastically clear declarations tell us that the idea of the asylum can survive the apparent destruction of the asylum as institution.

Last Things

The psychiatry possible today is the best of all possible psychiatries: this is the bequest Franco Basaglia has left us, and with the passing of years his achievement has only grown more impressive; however, psychiatry as he imagined and practiced it needs grand idealistic drive, a strong passion for hope, an ample clinical and psychopathological culture, and also a human one capable of drawing out its extraordinary therapeutic, scientific, and transformative potential. In any case, psychiatry has now taken another turn: the asylum superstructure has been removed from psychiatry, which now takes place in local and national hospitals and communities and is, at its core, an interpersonal and social psychiatry that nonetheless requires an idealistic impulse and an emotional and cultural rebirth, not only within psychiatry but on the part of the social and nursing staff that form an essential part of psychiatry in the public hospital. In the following part of this work, I will detail the essential thematic outlines of a psychiatry that renews and updates Basaglia's ideals.

IV. The Psychiatry of the Future

Psychiatry has entered public hospitals and is now part of the national health service, but a radical change and improvement in the structures and methods in psychiatric practice is insufficient if, as is the case today, exclusive importance is granted to pharmaceuticals to the detriment of therapies based on attention and listening, sensitivity and passion, emotional engagement, and the capacity to grasp the hidden meaning of psychic suffering, of madness, and the enormous importance of dialogue in treatment. *Homo faber, homo robot* rise up within us, in everyday life and in psychiatry, which is nonetheless inherently oriented toward relations, toward dialogue, toward giving the unwell person the time they need. Only if the psychiatry of the future manages to recover these values, of which my pages would like to reconstruct the essential lines, will the ideals that animate Basaglia's work be reborn, ideals that today are frequently overshadowed by a psychiatry consumed by the technicisms that are the epistemological core of the *DSM*.

The Heart of the Reform

The radical and earth-shattering consequence of the reform law was the closure of the asylums, and forty years after the fact, we must not forget the revolutionary significance of that act; but what is often neglected is the theoretical foundations of Basaglia's thought and work, which the psychiatry of the future should examine with extreme interest and with the Leopardian passion for hope that I previously invoked. The heart of this revolution in the way we practice psychiatry is reflected in Basaglia's writings: we psychiatrists are compelled to seek out a role we've never played before, one that allows us, insofar as possible, to place on to the level of those who are suffering in a space where illness, as a category, is set aside. Only in this way can one enter into an immediate relation of care with a person plagued by anguish and suffering, turmoil and despair, hallucinations and deliria, with the need to be taken in and assisted with respect for their pain and wounded dignity. I must reassert that asylum psychiatry did not vanish from the concrete behavior of no small number of psychiatrists, and continues in the form of an exclusive emphasis on illness to the detriment of a patient's interiority, subjectivity, and life story, ignoring the radical importance of the emotions in the understanding and amelioration of psychic suffering, considered not with the coldness of a surgeon who slices into an afflicted organ and sews it back together, but as an open, bleeding wound that must be treated with sensitivity and kindness, with compassion and introspection, with vigilant immersion in the life story of the sick person, necessarily the basis of a psychiatry open to the horizons of social psychiatry. Let me repeat: Basaglia's work cannot be properly understood separate from its phenomenological origins; and it is not the absence of structural alternatives to the asylum, or adequate forms of helping patients' families, that make it difficult to carry out the normative demands of the reform law, but rather the failure to value the ethical and social ideals that lie at its core.

These ideals, their realization, must be the focal point of any future psychiatry that aims to be humane and kind.

Ideal Goals

An ideal psychiatry must push for the elimination of restraints and electro-shock, which are cruel therapies for schizophrenia and depression, and must place its trust in a new generation of psychiatrists that will possess the drive and the imagination to rediscover and reconceive lost models of psychiatry that hearken back to radical changes of the previous generation. It is impossible to say exactly how to animate or envision this unfinished revolution, even if the path is traced out in the expectations and hopes, the concreteness and historicity, of the initiatives that Basaglia imagined and carried out. We need what I would call a complementary revolution, that restores passion and inspiration to the content of the law, to its extraordinary theoretical and practical implications, and that overcomes the indifference and inertia in contemporary psychiatry and public opinion, which has turned away from this subject while in the 1970s was widely supportive of closing the asylums. The political neglect of psychiatry, its human and social problems, has set aside and thus greatly weakened the ideals of the law, and it is to those that we must, perhaps updating their application to our new historical context but without adding on useless modifications or amendments that would distract from the burning problems yet to be solved. There are still psychiatric hospitals that keep patients behind locked doors and cold barred windows that accentuate their autistic isolation, and an excessive administration of pharmacological cocktails entirely removed from a relational context that is necessarily psychotherapeutic and sociotherapeutic.

To Not Forget

The dragon of forgetting has cruelly descended on the deserted asylums, those places of infinite pain and unspeakable loneliness. Ours is an age that lives in the present, forgetting the past and looking away from the future, which cannot but be interwoven with the past, as in that splendid image of Saint Augustine's that defines hope as the memory of the future. Psychiatry cannot be understood without reflecting on the abysses of pain that accompany psychic suffering, its loneliness, the isolation of asylums, which marked the days and nights of young and old alike, of young people who grew old, at times never moving from one place, one single place, even a chair, a single chair. Not all asylums were like this: Novara wasn't like this, I repeat, at least not in the women's section, where we were, for a time, able to recreate humane and gentle living conditions. It's true that the madness of women is better able to resist pain, how to release pain with more intense and creative emotions and words; and by giving words to pain, welcoming another person into it, means mitigating it, at least a little. The words of these patients are gathered in my books, and even if it is only for the very brief time of a morning, they were saved from catastrophe and silence. These are words that in my memory are connected to the tears and smiles, to the defenseless kindness and innocence of these patients. There were times when the asylum was this, too.

The memory of wounded spirits should be accompanied by the places they inhabited and experienced in pain and in hope against all hope, even if they are only present in the recollections of the people who have known them. These are places sealed by pain, that we should view with care and respect: as things marked by suffering. I repeat, these are things that should be presented and taught in schools, even in primary schools, in order to give an understanding of what psychic suffering is, what sensitivities and fragilities it feeds on, and how it can manifest in any of us. Only in this way—and this has occurred in some Austrian schools—can we defeat those still-rampant prejudices that see psychic suffering as a form of life foreign to the human condition and destitute of meaning, ignoring its kindness and tenderness, its loneliness and despair, its nostalgia for a smile and for a tear.

These are indications that can be understood in their radiant significance only if psychiatry is recognized and lived—in its technical and scientific facets, but also in its ethical ones, which the psychiatry of the future should try desperately to actualize in its complex and ardent human richness, which is irreconcilable with its reduction to a natural science.

Words in Psychiatry

Psychiatry has never given much importance to the words spoken to patients, showing no concern for the pain that indifferent and cruel language can cause. I have examined this subject in some of my works, but I would like to reformulate it briefly now with relation to a psychiatry projected from the past and present into a future interwoven with hope and directed toward respect for the fragility and dignity of madness. In rebuilding psychiatry ethically over the rubble of the asylums, the psychiatry of the future necessarily acquires immense importance, and we cannot cease thinking of it. And it is something the clinical psychiatric texts ignore, or if it is mentioned, it is dismissed as outdated and antiscientific. I would like again to highlight again its enormous diagnostic and therapeutic significance, and not only in psychiatry.

Hugo von Hofmannsthal, the great *fin-de-siècle* Austrian writer, tells us with extraordinary sensitivity and great psychological intuitiveness, that words are living creatures. They are born, modulated and modified, they change in our encounters in life, awakening highly diverse emotional connotations: sometimes serenity and joy, sometimes pain and grief. They are binding for those who utter them, and for those who listen to them, they change their meaning insofar as they change our mood, our emotions, and our passions. And so it is difficult to capture the resonances they trigger for us and others. Once spoken, they no longer belong to us, and they change in their arcane relation with the unspoken language of smiles and laughter, looks and gestures, and silence: because yes, even silence speaks, we must simply know how to listen to it, how to enter into its endless dialogue. The path of words, of the words we speak and those we hear, is a mystery. Words that are beautiful and creative in one context may not be so in another, and we must know how to recognize them in their light and shadow, their horizons open to hope and closed to it.

When psychiatry is confronted with complex experiences such as psychosis, there is even greater need for fragile and silent words that are capable of establishing relations of care. Without these words, it is impossible to delve into the infinite discourse of pain and anguish, sorrow and despair, turmoil of the heart and dread of the soul, voices and silence, that form part of every human suffering. In particular, the words spoken to a depressed, lost, desperate patient must synchronize with their way of experiencing time: such a person lives in the past, and the future slowly reemerges as the illness dissipates. Still more difficult are the words to be spoken to the patient stranded in the shadows of schizophrenia—of which there are, nevertheless, milder and more serious forms—which leave them sensitive to every word that is not kind and careful not to awaken uncertainty or the feeling of persecution. The psychiatry of the future ought not to consider futile or rhapsodic these apparent linguistic digressions which are unknown in asylum psychiatry and beyond.

Words That Don't Wound

We will never find the words that don't wound, that help those living in pain, unless we empathize with their emotions and relive them insofar as we are capable. There are no recipes, no recommendations in this field, one has to trust the subtle antennas of intuition and personal sensitivity. There are psychiatrists and psychologists who lack these, and regular people who have them: these antennas are innate, at least in part, though each of us can learn to develop them to some extent. We cannot communicate with psychic suffering unless we avoid words that are vague and banal, ambiguous and indifferent, glacial and abstract, cruel and anonymous. If we are not sad, or anxious, or disturbed, or desperate, words, even unhappy words, hardly touch us; but if we are, or if we have been, the emotional resonances of these words build painfully within us, leaving bleeding wounds that will not heal. If we are struggling, as we surely will at some point in our lives, we can never hear words like "insane," "crazy," "mental patient," "dangerous," or "senile" (flaunted with horrible blitheness at any failing of the memory of the elderly, who cannot escape this label, even in the absence of clinical dementia), without feeling pointlessly wounded in ways that sometimes will never heal.

These are words that harm even those who utter them, hollowing them from within.

Not Only in Psychiatry

As the great French oncologist David Khayat has written, words are enormously powerful: they can raise hope in a patient's heart, they are the gift of a humanity that the doctor must keep alive, to accompany his expertise, in his heart. He often encountered people hurt by words that were too harsh and inhumane, words spoken by their doctor. The words of a doctor, an oncologist or otherwise, are never neutral, are never muted or insignificant, and leave deep traces in patients suffering in a state of painful expectation. (I know such words cannot be found in psychiatric texts, but rather, for example, the letters of Mother Teresa of Calcutta). Not knowing what to say, or how to find the words that help, it is better, far better, to be silent, and to acknowledge pain with a simple clasp of the hand, which (alone) would have helped, to quote Paul Celan, one of the great German-language poets of the past century, who died of suicide in the waters of the Seine. The mysterious grace of intuition permits us to find the helpful words in the hour of pain and anguish, the words without which one cannot search for a psychiatry oriented toward the future.

This is a central subject of my considerations in this book: language, its dramatic importance in everyday life, a necessary tool in the psychiatry of the future, whose calling must be to bring humanity to lives of suffering and the various institutions devoted to its care.

Cristina Campo

The vast and chameleonic theme of words, their phenomenology and their thematic articulations, is endlessly analyzable in the human sciences or in psychiatry, which is one of them. Even in everyday life, we must carefully consider the words we use, assaying their resonances in others, and not forgetting that they have their own histories. The enigmatic and otherworldly words of Cristina Campo always speak profoundly to my imagination and my sense of hope. I don't know how many recognize the lightness and the vertiginous depth of the thought that is reflected in this quotation: "Every word is offered in its multiple meanings, like the strata of a geologic column: each one differently colored and differently inhabited, each one reserved for the reader whose intensity of attention will allow him to discern and decipher it. But for everyone, when a poem is pure, it comes as an abundant gift that is simultaneously partial and total: beauty and meaning independent yet inseparable, as in a communion." And, with extreme tenderness: "Everyone who heard the master speak, says a Hebrew tale, felt they were hearing a secret destined for his ears alone, and so everyone felt the marvelous story the master told in the squares belonged to him and was complete, although every newcomer heard only a fragment." Is this not a beautiful image, an arcane metaphor, of what happens, or could happen, when a mysterious consonance between speaker and listener whether a relation between two people or in a larger group to enter into a sort of shell where emotions and thoughts can be shared in silence and in acceptance? Can we not see clearly how the breath of mystery sometimes leads us, when we find ourselves in a state of grace, to intuit what the emotions of a person are even before they've been expressed? Are these not the intuitions that the great Dutch psychiatrist H.C. Rümke, among others, added to his diagnoses in his encounters with patients, perhaps from respect for that attention that Simone Weil said was a form of prayer? I am not sure, but I am certain the magic words of Cristina Campo are relevant to psychiatry, revealing its intuitive inner dimension that makes of every encounter, every dialogue, a challenge to cold reason. My wish is that the psychiatry of the future not forget the great importance, which today's psychiatry has vehemently denied, of phenomenological insight in our understanding of what is a normal or a pathological psychic life. Not all of psychiatry's past deserves to be erased or even demonized: that I cannot accept.

Listening

The words care requires can be found only if we are trained and habituated to listening, but how do we listen in psychiatry? I cannot forget the profound change in the women's asylum in Novara when we were there next to the patients, young and old, listening to them from one day to the next, helping to reawaken resources in them that had been forgotten but not lost. Today, however, we have less and less time to listen, asking questions oriented toward the cataloguing of symptoms and not the life history that gives those symptoms meaning.

There are countless forms of listening, but especially in psychiatry listening is impossible without keeping in mind the patient's expectations and hopes along with an awareness and sympathetic comprehension of their experience of inner time. How innumerable are our occasions to listen, yet how often are we capable of immersing ourselves in the thoughts and emotions of others, sick and well, that we encounter? How much suffering and how many wounds we would avoid if we persistently attempted to foresee what is happening in us, in our own interiority, and in that of others—their expectations, right or wrong, kept silent or shouted. Each day, we are assailed by expectations; those of the people we treat or care for who ask for help: the help of a word, a look, a gesture, a simple handshake, the help of the people from time to time life, everyday life, brings to us. It may be the expectant beggar who passes by whom we fail to greet, listen to, embrace: lost, perhaps, in the depths of a loneliness that our indifference strips of all hope, that Goethian shooting star without which it is impossible to live or even survive.

To hear the words of those who have known and emerged from suffering is necessarily one of the first steps on the path that the psychiatry of the future should take.

Scars

The shadow that lies next to us when we have known psychic suffering may never vanish, or it may grow thinner and thinner until it dissolves. The shadow born from psychotic and schizophrenic experiences never goes away, and becomes a scar that will never heal, when memories of the episode of illness reemerge in our memory and we cannot manage to rid ourselves of them. These aching memories sometimes linger in the river of mortal anguish and voluntary death.

The clinical categories of recovery and non-recovery are not easily adaptable to the complex and paradoxical reality of psychotic experiences in which the symptoms of illness, deliria and hallucinations may be necessary to the patient's survival, and it may be dangerous to dispel them pharmacologically because this clinical recovery might produce an unbearable vacuum. A solitary despair. It is better to fight the whole world than to be alone, as one of the great fathers of psychiatry in the German language of the last century wrote. The shadow that accompanies depression in its onset and progress attenuates as the illness improves, and when one is better, even its shadow disappears, but melancholy follows, a non-pathological mood which, like its Leopardian analogue, causes us to view the world with a bitter, painful nostalgia (I recommend Romano Guardini's indescribably beautiful and poignant writings on melancholy).

Fragility

Madness is fragile, as is timidity and sensitivity, and today there is a tendency to dismiss it. Yet this should never occur in the psychiatry of tomorrow, which proposes to stress its human and phenomenological dimensions. I will now reflect briefly on certain aspects of fragility that pertain to the major psychopathological experiences of depression and schizophrenia.

Fragility is a word whose vast semantic horizons touch on weakness, vulnerability, delicacy, and sensitivity, and is linked to madness. There are fashionable words that die no sooner than they are born, and there are others that fashion rescues from oblivion and that resist the passage of time, retaining their meaning and currency because they are dense with deep and indelible significance. Such, I believe, is the fate of fragility, even if there is not always a clear and adequate awareness of its complexity and its psychological and human meaning. There is a fragility that is shadow, a vague weariness with life, the dark night of the soul (pain, melancholy, madness), and there is a fragility that is grace, the luminous thread of life. And the two things overlap. Madness is fragile in its immense pain, and thus readily susceptible to the wounds of life, which we should respect and recognize in their dignity and in their longing to be heard and to dialogue, shedding the cruel prejudice that deems madness a useless experience.

Madness is fragile, but it allows us to grasp deep realities of the human condition that would otherwise remain hidden. Adolescence is fragile, with its conflicts with a society that doesn't know how to embrace its expectations and hopes; old age is fragile in its weakness and anguish, its desire to be heard and accepted. Fragility obliges us to consider the precariousness of our desires and our expectations; our hopes and our illusions: our lives. But how do we recognize our own fragility and that of others? Naturally, we must escape the feverish restlessness of our days with their frequent distractions from inwardness, and recover solitude, that great inner solitude that allows us to descend into the depths of ourselves, and has nothing to do with that isolation that is the counter-image of inner solitude.

It isn't easy to salvage solitude, that treasure island always sought after and in essence never found, though we never weary of searching for it. Solitude is a fine fellow traveler on the road of our lives, even if a painful one, because it confronts us with our emotions, our passions, our fragility, and our disappointments, which help us to understand those of others. We do not want this fragility inside us, and we are constantly tempted not to recognize it, to consider it an experience alien to our lives, something to be confined to areas of experience that don't pertain to us. Madness is the sign and emblem of fragility, extreme fragility, but also of solitude, of painful solitude, which longs for the light of a friendly word and a silent gaze. But life, as the great Austrian poet George Trakl says, devoured by solitude and by the search for voluntary death, echoes with harmonies and gentle madness.

The psychiatry of the future ought never forget fragility as a secret dimension of madness, nor the community of fate as a dimension of the treatment of madness in its yearning for dialogue and endless interrelation between healer and healed.

The Community of Fate

Things become complicated when one attempts to define the phenomenological roots of the community of fate that the psychiatry of tomorrow, called to eternally emphasize its human content, should be able to recover, by grafting it onto the truncated revolution Basaglia carried out in the spirit of a psychiatry distracted by entities incapable of recognizing the deep significance of madness and treating it humanely.

What can we say, then, of the community of fate, which is not a utopia but an attainable goal based on the phenomenological understanding of psychic life? The community of fate is there when we feel the fate of pain, anguish, suffering, despair, joy and hope, of the other who is with us as though it were, at least in part, our fate as well. What is required here is the creation of a community of fate by immersing ourselves in the emotional world of the patient, trying to recognize and value, insofar as possible, its extreme inward tensions of anguish, sorrow, and despair. The community of fate is visible to the eyes of the heart, though, and not to the cold gaze of Cartesian reason. A therapeutic community can only exist in the horizon of a community of fate as reborn in the conscience of each of us, and in the relations we have with others: in the family, in school, in care work, in labor in its various forms. To recognize oneself in the fragile destiny of another means, among other things, to keep this fragility present in understanding those behaviors which reveal their nuances of meaning beneath its light. Only by moving from our interiority, by immersing ourselves in our emotional life, is it possible to follow the words, the words of hope and silence, the words of listening and dialogue, that allow the person who is ill, their antennas of suffering highly sensitive, to find themselves in a condition of acceptance and human salvation. Fate, the fate of pain and anguish, of sorrow and despair, becomes a painful life experience that is salvaged in its horizons of meaning when it meets with a word, a look, a smile, a tear that comes from the heart.

There are communities of souls wounded by life, communions of fates that are reborn in the depths of lives consumed nowadays by quite different challenges: floodlights that never turn off, doggedly pursued success, riches flaunted and concealed, indifference to the reasons of the heart and insensitivity to pain and sacrifice. There are communities that cross over from psychiatry into sociology, and from our common form of earthly life into actions and sites of salvation (for example, the rare and glorious testimony of Mother Teresa).

The Great Communitarian Movements

The psychiatry of the future must foresee or be aware of the deep changes in society, those that are now evident and those that will take place in the coming years and make it even more fragile. I will say a few words about them now.

The great communitarian movements, which are gradually withering away, marked the 1960s and 70s, when culture, even political culture, was highly sensitive to the anguish of life in the asylums and the harsh wounds inflicted on the dignity and freedom of patients who lived in conditions of cruel dehumanization: in the vast majority of asylums, though not in all of them, people were dying of loneliness. Those were years when asylums revealed their unprecedented abnegation of every right and all respect for persons, and the scandal and moral revolt were such that people's conscience, the conscience of civil society, became indignant. Today, things have changed, and the psychiatry of the future will no longer be able to count on these great vital movements, and must become aware of the faults of the community and society and not be submerged by them.

The dominant climate is one of indifference to the values of solidarity and empathy with the suffering of others, psychic suffering in particular. We feel increasingly alone, we are increasingly alone, ever more abandoned, ever more prone to the fear that others will not listen to us and will not concern themselves with our fate, and the situation is all the more grave when we are ill, disturbed, depressed, when psychic suffering descends upon us. The feeling grows that suffering lacks human meaning, and is seen as a source of guilt, something that, if we truly wanted to, we could get over and suppress.

Indifference is a cruel and cold affliction of psychic life, imprisoning us in the desert of hopelessness, which permits no real communication, no sincere relations, with the world or with things. In indifference, we are submerged in an arid and petrified solitude that has nothing to do with that creative inner solitude, but is simply isolation. In isolation, we become monads without doors or windows: all altruistic impulses frustrated, we are frozen in the glaciers of radical individualism. In indifference, all possible desire for community is snuffed out—community, which is the expression, the image, the living, palpable metaphor of a life worth living even in pain and suffering, in anguish and despair. Will the psychiatry of the future, its past rooted in phenomenology, its present in the revolution of 1978, be able to remain true to the structural renewal the law has brought about while bringing to fruition those ideals that constitute its backbone?

This is the hope born and not yet dead in the heart of those who knew the psychiatry of the past in its highest moments, which were real, along with that of the present, which has broken down walls that seemed untouchable and indestructible, rebuilding bridges that have changed the face of the world.

Madness

The final section of this chapter I would like to dedicate to madness, to the phenomenology of madness, which is a subject of psychiatry in all its forms, however variously it is described and defined, with an account of the life and death of two young women, one depressed, the other schizophrenic, so that whoever reads this book may witness the endless horizons of anguish and pain and sorrow and despair, but also of kindness and delicacy, fragility and shattered hope, that exist in madness, even if psychiatry has often shown itself unable to grasp these stories, and has instead ground to dust. I met one of these patients in the asylum and one of them outside it, and both show how madness is intertwined with deeply human forms of suffering; I would not like the psychiatry of the future ever to forget them in its task of not allowing it to suffocate, submerged in the endless cascades of technique in its multiple expressions. These are just two patients, but their symptoms mirror the essence of two emblematic psychopathological experiences, the depressive and the schizophrenic, which are conceptually interwoven with others that I have described in my writings over the course of many years and workplaces. They are intended to serve as human and clinical testimony, giving a soul to pages previously focused on methodological and theoretical questions.

The Wounds of the Soul

Psychiatry concerns itself not only with pathological depressions, depressions that require pharmaceutical intervention, but, I insist, with depressions that are a part of every person's life, of the lives of all of us who need healing words and to open our hearts to hope, which we must go in search of, and not simply drugs, which are not always useful.

What can we say to a patient rent with pain, pain of the soul and body, so often interwoven, when they ask us desperately for help? The words aren't easy to find, and sometimes we cannot find them, but a gesture, a caress, a smile, a tear, may dispel or at least lighten the shadows of suffering. I learned this well in the university clinic in Milan, in the asylum in Novara, in psychiatric services at the Ospedale Maggiore in Novara, and when I left, I was still able to accompany some of my patients along their path. But in this book, devoted to reflections on theoretical and practical aspects of psychiatry, I would like to say something about the life stories of two patients, one depressed, the other schizophrenic: Chiara and Margherita—from whose poetry I quoted earlier— who speak of the sensitivity and kindness, the fragility and delicacy, easily forgotten and ignored by clinical psychiatry today. But what of the lacerating presence of pain, the pain invisible to the indifferent and distracted eyes of a psychiatry concerned only with symptoms, with depressive or hallucinatory and depressive symptoms, coldly taken apart and put back together, and not with the interiority of patients, the interiority that bleeds from the painful wounds of Chiara and Margherita. A testimony of pain and anguish nearly unseen, nearly forgotten, in a psychiatry that has as its only educational text the various editions, already mentioned, of the *DSM*, in particular its fifth edition, in which there is no importance placed on pain, human suffering, inner life, the emotional resonances of illness, as if they didn't matter, as if they weren't prerequisites to healing; no mention of the carefully chosen words and gestures, the smiles and tears, that form part of treatment, whether in a community of care or a community of fate. We are not dealing with illnesses that can be treated with the cold and autonomous administration of antidepressant, anti-anxiety, anti-psychotic (neuroleptic) drugs; we are dealing with people who are extremely sensitive to the words they hear and the comprehension of their suffering, their expectations, and their shattered hopes. What useful and humane psychiatry—a natural science but also, perhaps above all, a human one, a science of the spirit as the German language defines it—can be practiced if there is no attention to the wounded humanity, the pain in patients' souls; a wounded humanity such as the one Chiara and Margherita attest to. I would like their words to be pondered here and not forgotten.

Chiara

This is Chiara: a young mother who lost her only child at ten years old. Her life lost all meaning, the days were all equal, they began and ended without leaving a trace. She worked as a teacher in a nursery school in contact with many children that reminded her endlessly of her own, and the love she devoted to them was the only thing that kept her alive in the solitude of a home sunken deeper and deeper in the silence of the heart and an aching nostalgia for the impossible. What could I say to this young mother wracked with unspeakable pain, who had lost all hope and sense of expectation? I sat in silence, never looking at the clock, its hands still turning with no regard for her pain, as she yearned for that prayer that is attentive listening (again Simone Weil's ineffable, radiant phrase) that would allow this patient—I call her that, but in the face of a misfortune such as Chiara's, who wouldn't be one?—to give voice to her despair. In the slow hours of a therapy session, which seemed never-ending in its openness and closure to an indescribable hope, I tried to empathize with Chiara's chasms of pain and anguish, which I would regard in silence with that fragile and torn gaze that would allow me to recognize them.

I cannot help but think of the enigmatic and luminous words of Giovanni Pozzi in that book of such striking beauty, *Tacet*, where he speaks of silence in ways that help me grasp its mysterious and delicate composition. "To listen, one must be silent, not only keep a physical silence that refrains from interrupting the speech of others (or if it does, it resumes immediately thereafter to continue listening) but an inner silence, a disposition oriented entirely to the reception of another's words. It is necessary to silence the commotion of one's own thoughts, still the restlessness of the heart, the tumult of stress, every sort of distraction. Nothing can make clearer the correlation between silence and words as listening, true listening."

A silence like this, a silence that can hear the beating of hearts, both one's own and that of the person seeking our help, is what we require when fate presents us with a young mother like Chiara whom an arid psychiatry with its classifications and diagnoses would simply send back to the depression clinic for its consequent pharmacological treatment. How can one think that antidepressants could be at all helpful in relieving the immense pain and the infinite solitude that tormented Chiara's soul? When we encounter patients like these in psychiatry, who are drowning in sorrow and suffering, in the loss of all hope, the only way forward is constant listening, allowing ourselves to be affected by the things that they say, even when following them down the mysterious path to our inner depths isn't easy. I don't know if practicing psychiatry is even possible, with a patient like Chiara, without creating a community of healing that opens up into a community of fate, one reflected in the vulnerable if rare figure of kindness.

Kindness Again

There is no treatment, whether of body or soul, that is not accompanied by shreds of kindness that allow psychiatrists to find their patients in the horizon of mutual understanding. There is no kindness not born from the heart of interiority, from the knowledge that we are all summoned to the common fate of dignity and solidarity. It's true that these words seem to come from another world, the world of nostalgia and utopia, and yet the radical changes that have taken place in Italian psychiatry grew out of this kindness, this dialogical receptiveness to the other, these expectations, these hopes. Kindness opens us to the moods and sensitivities of others, to the suffering in particular, and to interpret cries for help that come not only from their words, but also from their eyes and their expressions. Kindness is like a bridge that brings healer and healed into mysterious contact; but it is also a bridge because it pulls us out from the confines of ourselves, our subjectivity, and makes us participants in the inner life, the subjectivity, of others, of patients, creating invisible alliances, invisible communities of fate that ease the stranglehold of loneliness and suffering. There is no form of care of the body or the spirit that does not attend to such moods and ways of being as kindness, tenderness, humility, and intelligence of the heart, which overlap not only in psychiatry but also in life. Clinical practice, with its quick and abrupt time scale does not always permit the emergence of these forms of life into the living flesh of a therapeutic conversation, and yet we are all called, each in our own way, to find in ourselves the treasure island of kindness and humility where we must touch ground, and from which we move to give a hand to cruel and imponderable fates like Chiara's. One cannot do otherwise if one wants to keep alive the hope, that fugitive shooting star, that is in us and above all in the person shipwrecked on the rocks of immeasurable pain.

(We should never forget Friedrich Hölderlin's unfathomable and memorable words about kindness as the goal to strive for in life within a horizon of hope that does not fade even in the most extreme situations of life. "As long as kindliness, which is pure, remains in his heart not unhappily a man may compare himself with the divinity. Is God unknown? Is He manifest as the sky? This rather I believe. It is the measure of man. Full of acquirements, but poetically, man dwells on this earth. But the darkness of night with all the stars is not purer, if I could put it like that, than man, who is called the image of God.")

In the heart of psychiatry is the relation, the intersubjectivity that stems from kindness and humility, fragile and dialogical emotions, rooted in the horizons of meaning of clinical and social psychiatry alike: two images, each interwoven with the other, of a shared psychopathological and human reality.

Margherita

From Chiara, the Leopardian and Schubertian image of a deeply human depression that would be better called melancholy or vital sorrow, I would now like to move on to Margherita, the image of a much deeper psychic suffering characterized by that form of dissociation which is the basic structure of schizophrenia: a word which even today evokes anguish and despair and should be banished from psychiatry, but cannot be, and feeds on the same human anguish and suffering that I cannot forget even at a distance of so many years. I met Margherita, a young mother, as I recall, in the asylum, our unusual women's asylum in Novara, and I described her life and her poetry in my book *The Poetic Experience of a Schizophrenic.* I would like to turn back to this book, written in 1971, seven years before the passage of the psychiatric reform law, to describe the kindness, sensitivity, and deeply human suffering possible in psychotic conditions like schizophrenia, the humanity of which is unjustly negated, as well as the complexity, the thorniness, the difficulty, the pain that accompanies its treatment, which the reform law made possible throughout Italy, but which was not altogether new in a humane asylum such as ours. We cannot talk about social psychiatry without keeping in mind the human dimension and the consequent infinite importance of listening and of dialogue with the unquiet, wounded soul of madness and of women's madness in particular. We mustn't let ourselves be deceived by the symptoms of the illness, delusions and hallucinations, or emotional disturbances that were present in Margherita, for they also carried a sensitivity and a creative imagination that can still stir the heart today. Obviously, it doesn't matter whether anyone remembers my words, those words from a time so long ago reevoked in this book now, but I hope—my slight, delicate hope—that the dragon of forgetting will not utterly erase Margherita's painful and poetic words. One cannot speak of psychiatry, as I constantly repeat, much less a cognitively and therapeutically advanced psychiatry, that does not include listening to patients, or a psychiatry of the future that does not attend to their human experiences of suffering and hope.

The Other World

Margherita was twenty-five years old when she entered the asylum after episodic hallucinations and delirium accompanied by, sunken as she was in the dark waters of agony, thoughts of suicide, which persisted intermittently for five years. The doctor, offering her a cigarette, seemed to have hatred in his eyes, she thought that the cigarette was laced, and she was filled with painful anxiety: "Everyone is against me. I don't understand why there's so much hate against me. I don't see this hate from you, at least for now, but it could happen. It's a question of sensibility. I know what I'm saying sounds absurd to you; if I heard this from another person, I wouldn't believe it either. But I know what I've experienced." Her discomfort increased despite antipsychotic drugs, and Margherita's world became filled with terror. "Yesterday some people came to ask me for a basin, and it was to collect my blood. They'll gouge out my eyes, they'll cut off my legs and make it look like an accident." These are fragments of the hallucinatory, delirious thinking she was submerged in, and led to a few months in the asylum, and was eventually discharged on high doses of medication. A psychotic condition was undeniably present, a schizophrenia characterized by delirious and hallucinatory shifts in meaning, an autistic solitude that permitted no interaction between her and others; and yet, what wounded gentleness was there, what human sensitivity in Margherita's emotional life, which was only apparently barren and petrified. We forget these things easily when we find ourselves with patients consumed by hallucinations and deliria, apparently bereft of all emotional impulse, not infrequently administered pharmaceuticals without a thought to the words spoken to them in the belief that they are pointless—so they say. Her poetry is a beautiful testament to this inner emotional richness.

Her Poetry

In the years between twenty-two and twenty-five years of age, Margherita composed strikingly beautiful poetry that attested to her sensitivity and abundant humanity. Her poems were written amid shattering deliria and hallucinations, and I would like to cite them in their remarkable variety. Beyond their lyrical suggestiveness, these poems confirm what some of the great psychiatrists of the past century always maintained, and that is worth repeating here: that psychosis and schizophrenia do not signify the extinction of the emotions, and that these people continue to live in ways filled with human significance, perhaps creative significance. These poems speak to us of pain, of bitter pain, of pain in the soul and in the body: for Chiara, this was accompanied by depressive symptoms, and in Margherita by psychotic and schizophrenic ones, and I always insist that when we encounter patients like these, consumed by deliria and hallucinations and imprisoned in autistic solitude, we must take into account the traces of unfathomable pain that are never absent.

I would like to add to the burning, indescribably painful poetry I cited previously other poems that bring us into the limitless thematic latitudes of Margherita's poetic experience.

The first of these is colored by the shadows of painful nostalgia that does not terminate in arid despair, but is interwoven with the shooting stars of a fragile and audacious hope that leads her to aspire to an almost impossible joy of living, expressed in the wounded tenderness of the final verses:

I would like to remain in time
Unpicked agave
Stuck in this land.

The gnarled souls of the olive trees in the wind
Radiate out
In dusty caresses
Remnants of sky and stars.

And lying on this field in August
I want to be the joy of life.

The forest goes up in flame
Of dry needles,
Of solar broom,
And from the arboreal grates of the olive trees
A soft light filters through
Kindling the stones
Like shards of ice
Against the sky.

And the flavor of life returns.

The day
In long flights and drowsy chatter
Is lost at sea.
Dawn comes to the shore
And with the clear skies
The gulls.

The second of these poems thematizes the disconsolate resignation to the meaninglessness of life.

There are people without smiles
With empty eyes
Faces without joy

Who obtusely live
Their everyday lives.

People without history
Without ideas, without love
Or compassion.

Dawns useless for them
Hearts still and calm
Hearts of stone
Hearts of indifference.

And life passes in its grayness,
It doesn't ask and doesn't give.

The eye darkens
Words are gaunt
Gestures ragged
Pride and humility are gone.

What remains is obtuse indifference
To appease the spirit
For our own uselessness.

The third poem is marked by the burning flames of a painless lament that haunts wounded Margherita's soul, wrapped up in the secret fascination of a love that seems unrequited despite her ardent prayer.

It was already a time for memories.
My spirit like a granary.

Pitchforks in hay.
Corn by the walls.

Slow millraces in swirls of fog.
Blue-hued moor.

And the days drifted away...
Thicket of shrubs to burn.

I stayed awake
On rainy starless nights,
And the light found me
Humbled and defeated,
Face dry from a painless lament.

And without life and without regrets
I waited in time.

Then you arrived,
No love, which means nothing at all,
But I gave you my hand,
A hinted prayer that you would stay.

...For I've long known the flavor of my frugal meal.

A fourth poem is suffused with a fatalistic and aching nostalgia for death that eventually becomes voluntary death. These are heartfelt and elegiac words that can never be read without emotion.

I will die at dawn
On a day like this.
The pallid sun will rise in rays
Behind the moor.

Assembled swallows will fly.
[...]

Face tranquil
eyes open to a seagull's flight
Over the green October sea.

[...]
A memory of geraniums and agaves
On a narrow Ligurian street.

[...]
Mother's tears
And I will be no more.

My humble years
Will lap at my things
In my old house,
Tragic nest.

The glass of the surrounding wall
Will wound my racing soul.
[...]

When I am dead
Put me in a white bridal dress.
It will not clash with my sincere eyes.

Take me to the seaside
To the fresh air
Laughing with Mediterranean flowers.
Take me far from the canals and ditches
That languish in this sad plain.

Carry me in a wicker basket
The kind that kids use
To steal figs

And do not weep

For from the bell tower
I will watch you
Smiling and white.

The anguish of death seems to dissolve into the musical rhythm of verses, but this is only an appearance.

What Else to Say

Margherita's poetic experience, beyond any aesthetic evaluation, must be heard in terms of its painful, rending message, which compels us to reflect again on the dimensions, not only psychopathological but also human, of psychiatric illness, and the importance within it of words and gestures, silence and the language of the face, with which we approach patients immersed in the flames of psychic suffering. Who, when reading this poetry, can help but feel anguish at the emotional impulses born of the burning bushes of psychosis?

In the years afterward, periods of alternating remission and relapse in a life that allowed Margherita to teach at a secondary school while continuing with her psychotherapy and her neuroleptic and anti-anxiety drugs. I cannot forget her fragility and her immense suffering. She wasn't unaware of her illness, indeed, its presence was acute and painful for her, she was mauled by deliria and hallucinations that made a normal life impossible, and she sometimes relived them as the consequence of a personal guilt she couldn't escape from, and that at times consumed her. I remember the relentless grinding past of the months when she was ill and painful thoughts of suicide recurred to her, and the months when she was well, and hope was her life's luminous companion, and everything changed within her and around her. The deliria and hallucinations disappeared, the barriers that isolated her so radically from the world of people and things collapsed, and Margherita was able to emerge from her radical autistic solitude. Toward the end of her life, we lost sight of her, and just before turning forty, when she was a patient in a hospital ward, not a psychiatric one, she died by suicide.

Pain as Leitmotif

In all my work, I have continually described and analyzed the life stories of those destiny has brought before me, but in this book, which has broader theoretical perspectives on the horizons of meaning in psychiatry, I wanted to base my discourse on the living fabric of the clinic through examples of depression, so frequent today, and of schizophrenic psychosis, which is much less frequent and nonetheless paradigmatic of diseases that may require the administration of those neuroleptic or antipsychotic drugs that have radically transformed courses of care that may lead to recovery.

These two patients, with their unusual tendency to introspection and to the narrativization of their sufferings and their experiences, reflect as through a mirror darkly the nature of anguish and sorrow, spiritual uncertainty and despair, their lives wounded by misfortune and a loss of meaning. These young patients' stories also reflect possible avenues of treatment, which can never be only pharmaceutical but must also be psychotherapeutic, with an emphasis on language, both of words and of the living body: of faces and looks, eyes and hands, tears and smiles. And I cannot avoid reiterating how the account of these two patients illustrates the importance in psychiatry, in its various symptomatological expressions within depression and psychosis, the experience of pain and suffering that Margherita's poetry makes plain in heartbreaking words we should never forget.

The Image of Madness

I would like to move now from these two young women immersed in the waves of mysterious and harrowing psychological suffering to the human image of madness, whose thematic horizons contain emotions marked by the vertigo of pain and anguish, hope and despair, shadow and light, and sometimes of the fatal yearning for voluntary death as the final expression of a cascade of illusions destroyed by life and fate. These emotions form part of life, everyday life and psychopathological life, but they can also lead to illness, flare up or die down, and they testify to the throbbing vitality of souls wounded by suffering and anguish. These are emotions which, I again stress, reveal themselves in their radically human and psychological dimensions only when rational consciousness is joined to an awareness born of the Pascalian reasons of the heart. The heart in flames as a living metaphor brings us close to the secret cipher of the human condition, a condition also distinguished by madness. Madness is not something extraneous to life, it is a human possibility within each of us, with its shadows and its emotional incandescence. The distance, the separation between psychotic and non-psychotic life is sometimes only quantitative, not qualitative. Sorrow and anguish are human experiences all of us are familiar with, and as Kurt Schneider, one of the great psychiatrists of the past century, once wrote, woe to those who haven't known them. It is only when they grow, when they burn, when they spread cruelly inside us, that sorrow and anguish become illnesses requiring pharmacological treatment. May we then banish completely the image of madness as one of the forms of life associated with insignificance, the incapacity to feel, insensitivity, indifference to values, aggressivity, and the perennial commonplace of violence. Madness is not violence, and to the extent that it becomes violent, it does so less frequently than normal life conditions. Finally, madness brings us face-to-face, as the life stories of Chiara and Margherita show painfully, with hidden and ignored aspects of humanity.

This endless river that is life, this river we are immersed in every day, sweeps us away and does not always allow us to reflect on what is hidden in its deep waters, which are the waters of our interiority; and when the shadows of psychological suffering descend on us, the waters of life's river stop, and there emerge from them amplifications of very significant human experiences. I have indicated a few of these: guilt and illness, sadness and anguish, that solitude that grades into autistic isolation, expectation and shattered hope, inner time that withers into the past and has no future before it, death and dying that loom with strange enchantment and linger almost immovably in the lives of depressives, so that their final hopes are placed in death itself.

I am aware of the immense sufferings of body and soul that madness brings with it, which may lead to the abysses of unspeakable despair, but even in situations such as these, life continues to attest to its human significance and to its worth however much, in a not so distant past, this was crudely questioned not only in public opinion, but in the psychiatry of the foregoing century. My hope is that the psychiatry of the future will never cease to reflect on the phenomenological and human dimensions, and not only on the clinical and psychopathological ones, of madness, which the psychiatry of the past and to a certain extent of the present has not managed or wished to recognize, thus failing to adapt to the necessary modes of listening and of care.

Final Reflections

Flashbacks

In these final pages, I would like to reflect on certain of the themes I have developed in the course of my book, which may yet spark fragile but not labile emotional consonances.

Dialogue, the search for dialogue, with madness as the leitmotif of my discourse here, has taken place in what I hope is an apotheosis of human intimacy, fostered by listening and acceptance, solitude and silence. In everyday life, but especially in dialogue with madness, we should never confront another, above all when the other is ill or asking for help, with an attitude of cold clinical distance and icy observation. None of us can truly know whether we remain only ourselves and are not at the same time another; and in knowing ourselves and in knowing others, we must follow the mysterious path that leads into our depths, as Augustine's admirable words reflect: *in interiore homine habitat veritas*. Following phenomenology, phenomenology experienced as a passion for difference, as Moritz Geiger writes (I read this definition in a beautiful letter sent to me by Gabriele Scaramuzza), in search of the madness that is also within us, in the splendid words of Kurt Schneider, I cannot avoid laying great clinical and diagnostic stress on emotional awareness, on the intuition that takes us down those perhaps dark and mysterious paths to anguish and sorrow, turmoil and aggression, solitude and despair, hallucinations and deliria, estrangement, which are the thematic domains of psychiatry: a psychiatry of the interior that endlessly rediscovers the human in madness. Phenomenology, my interpretation of phenomenology, has led me to grant epistemological and dialogical value to the language of words, those living creatures that can heal the wounds of body and soul or make them bleed endlessly, and can build bridges of communication with those people lost in the shadows of pain. But words are not enough to forge a therapeutic relationship if they are not infinitely interwoven with the language of silence and of the living body.

The Language of Silence

Every silence has a language, and it is not always easy to decipher its meanings, whether in everyday life or in psychology. How many times, in a therapeutic encounter, is a patient walled in by fragile silence that must not be broken by blithe, prying words that would cause harm. We must distinguish that silence which arises from a desire for solitude from the one that springs from deep depression that approaches the edges of an always possible voluntary death. We must also distinguish the silence that possesses a scintilla, a drop, of hope from the silence that emerges from our incapacity to hear hope's secret origins. Only words uttered from silence can sometimes save a life adrift, and psychiatry cannot disdain words and silence. It is difficult, when dealing with the burning bushes of obsession, depression, and schizophrenia, to choose when to speak and when to be silent, when to ask questions and when to give answers. Only intuition and education in emotional awareness can help us to choose what to say on the difficult path of treatment; and if we do not reflect on these questions, we will not find models of treatment adequate to the diverse forms of psychic suffering.

(Giovanni Pozzi's reflections on silent and solitude glimmer with such grace and beauty that I would like to cite them again here. "The cell and the book are rooms of solitude and silence. The cell of solitude is not a house of sticks in the desert, nor a walled prison, but lies at the center of man: the heart that never sleeps, vigilant in listening, a pure metaphor for the enclosed space and metonymy of the entire human person." And again, "From silence, the book, repository of memory, antidote to the chaos of oblivion, where the word lies sleepless, ready to make itself known with silent step to those who solicit it. A discreet friend, the book is not petulant, responds only when requested, does not urge beyond when asked to pause. Filled with words, it is silent." This is an audacious quote, it's true, but this book, like all my books, lives on the images and words, the pain and sorrow, the shattered hopes of my patients, and so this book is also theirs in its solitude and its silence).

The Hermeneutic Inquiry of Psychiatry

Psychiatry is an ambiguous and fraught discipline which, when it opens to the interdisciplinary horizon of research, not only looks into illnesses (psychic disturbances) but also confronts the phenomena of the world, their normal and pathological parts and in particular the endless archipelagos of the emotions. If, in practicing psychiatry, we are incapable of immersing ourselves in the inner life of others, particularly others who are unwell, if we are incapable of intuition (unable to draw on the fragile and ardent vessels of emotional consciousness that accompany rational consciousness), then it will be impossible to grasp the deeper sense of pain and suffering, sorrow and anguish, loss and the wounds of the soul, silence and the bewilderment of the heart that form part of the human condition in its infinite forms of expression in the normal and less-normal cases, which grade infinitely into each other.

These are the sources of my pages on the psychiatry of yesterday, today, and tomorrow, its possible clinical, psychopathological, phenomenological, and human variations; on memory and fear, on death and dying, on voluntary death as an excruciating human experience never alien to life; on the emotions, on sorrow and melancholy, on anguish and shattered hope, which glow, among other things, in the pain of certain poetic experiences.

The Common Thread of the Emotions

What are the common roots of the four parts that make up this book? In essence, the thesis that psychiatry is not only a natural science, but also a human one, which in caring for wounded interiorities follows cognitive paths fostered by kindness and sensitivity, ethics and humanity, helping to probe subject areas only seemingly foreign to psychiatry, while actually close to it in their common emotional background. Wounded emotions form part of depression, both monopolar and bipolar, pathological anxiety, and schizophrenia, though the last of these involves radical dissociation. Emotions accompany our lives not only amidst malaise, but in every circumstance, regardless of our wishes, whether we're ill or well, whether we're aware or not. My emotions, my experiences, changed when I was faced with depression or anxiety at the University Clinic in Milan, at the psychiatric hospital, and in Psychiatric Services at the Ospedale Maggiore della Carità in Novara, and the emotions of the patients in these conditions of treatment and life changed as well. Emotions, which accompanied me in their dizzying swings and turbulent fluctuations, are essential to memory's way of being, not only with its deep and at times unhealable wounds, as in Alzheimer's, but also in the normal conditions of life. The emotions are interwoven with fear, and with extreme knots, and how can we not perceive them as tumultuous and uncanny in the experiences of death and dying, especially with voluntary death? The common thread of emotions has woven through the light and shadow from the first page of this book in search of the paths hidden in everyday life that are ripe for rediscovery.

Today, philosophy and psychiatry are engaged in reassessing the importance of emotion in understanding psychological and human reality, and we cannot dispense with the emotions if we want to grasp the constituent structures of each of our inner lives. At any rate, one cannot practice psychiatry without looking at what Ingeborg Bachmann, the great Austrian writer, whose life was consumed by unpredictable surges of angst, considered the emblematic expressive distinction of Robert Musil's work: how his bitter and luminous words brought to the surface, and transformed into images, the deepest experiences of the soul.

Sorrow of the Soul in Poetry

I could not conclude the last part of this book devoted to psychiatry as hermeneutic inquiry, aimed at grasping the meaning of some of life's great themes, without reflecting on the sorrow of the soul and on melancholy. I do so by summoning images, metaphors, appearances, symbols, such as those that arise out of pain and torment but profound humanity as well in the poetry of Georg Trakl. We read it stunned and fascinated by the dizzying scale of emotions that runs from sweet and tender melancholy, fragile and submissive, silent and impalpable, evanescent and timid, to a biting and scarlet melancholy, febrile and stormy, cruel and stony, sometimes hallucinatory, sometimes intoxicating. These emotions, these emotional resonances, yield perhaps better to the timid, skittish gaze of psychiatry than to the academic and formal one of literary criticism that cannot quite manage to assimilate them or at least keep them present in its diverse and panoramic horizons of meaning. The goal of psychiatry can only be to arrive at an interpretation of the emotional contents of poetry and novels read with attention and listened to in a way different from clinical psychiatry. In all sorrow and melancholy (the semantic fields of the two overlap), the passage of time becomes wrinkled: the present impinges constantly on the past, which grows like a river with no reservoir to flow into, and the future crumbles and dies, no longer permitting hope to give meaning to life.

Trakl's poetry reminds us how numerous clinical layers underlie melancholy and life sorrow. As a mood, melancholy is a non-pathological emotional condition that overlaps with the sister experiences of sorrow, nostalgia, life distress, and depression, which is both near to and far from it, as a radicalization of sorrow in which its horizons of meaning expand vertiginously into an absence of future, or a future defined solely in terms of an anguish rendered thematic in the shadows of a past that swells, filled with guilt at transgressions never committed. In these poems, the boundaries between sorrow, melancholy, sweet melancholy, and depression, bitter and painful depression, shift from one to the next.

Pain

These pages of mine, which took as their ideal psychiatry as a form of life, as a destiny, are fundamentally marked by a common horizon of meaning: the encounter with pain, the pain of body and soul, with sadness and anguish, fears and fading memory, with fragility and silence, my sadness and my anguish, the longing for death and its feverish pursuit, which is the most aching and mysterious, rending and unpredictable subject of psychiatry, all psychiatry, beyond its assorted epistemological and therapeutic premises. Pain, an infinitely excruciating pain, is the thematic core of madness and any discourse about madness, and pain has been present to me, wounded, throbbing, and alive, in these pages, even beyond the thematic reconstruction of my life experiences. We should think always of pain, of that horrible and indescribable expression of it which is madness, speaking of it with fear and trembling whenever we psychiatrists and non-psychiatrists come across it—the madness of yesterday, of today, and of tomorrow, which the 1978 reform law allows to approach and treat in the best possible way.

Nostalgia

The heroes of this book are my patients, those from the past and those who continue to find the meaning of a listening that is unharmed by distraction or inattention, by the trivialization of pain, by the icy coldness of the soul. These patients accompanied me from the faraway years of the old asylum to those at the Ospedale Maggiore in Novara to today at the bulwark of clinic boldly facing the sheer, high mountain, Monte Rosa, with its perennial snow and its arcane and indecipherable silence. Nostalgia is not foreign to the fragile and brittle *Stimmung* that flows through these pages, unifying, I would like to hope, its narrative tones. Nostalgia is an infinite matrix of lost memories, and even fear can be mitigated by the intermittent lights of nostalgia, to which it is so difficult to escape in the hours of silence and reflection on the ineffable mystery of life. Perhaps this book with its zigzagging themes and its evolution may gather its arcane meanings in seasons sealed by silence and twilight, by shadows that descend on the heady glow of summer days.

Hopes

Thus ends a book, with its many thematic byways, that has tried to reconstruct my life in its infinite dialogue with psychiatry which, in the vertiginous passing of years, has changed the ways and the places of its practice. The image of psychiatry has changed, its modes of treatment have changed, but what didn't change was madness, psychic suffering in its fragility and its enigmatic origins. There is not only one psychiatry, but many, confronting our multiform experiences and visions of the world. But beyond all theoretical and cultural differences, psychiatry cannot exist without recuperating the inner meaning of humility and respect when faced with the sufferings of those afflicted by madness, and here, all of us should recognize ourselves beyond our individual destinies. Psychiatry cannot be practiced, perhaps, except with hope, the Kierkegaardian passion for the possible that is record and can be reborn even from the ashes of life conditions that appear lost, invulnerable to future change in the cold light of reason, but for which an apparently impossible rebirth is possible.

This is a book different from the many others I've written, perhaps because it is interwoven with fragments of my life, rhapsodic and winding, where experiences near and far in time have flowed together, faint and photographic descriptions, painful and brutal anecdotes, literary digressions and reflections deriving from a passionate, never concluded, ethos, a nostalgia for a time now extinguished by life, and for a psychiatry of ideals to which my destiny was anchored that seems to be in its death throes. But the hope for a psychiatry that does not wither in the arid deserts of technicism, and that retains awareness of the extreme humanity that shines in madness, can never die.

Answers

A question contains its answer, which is the same as my own. The mysterious path of nostalgia leads us to look into the abysses of a past where we reencounter the sources of what could have been our expectations and hopes, and they are revived: influencing whatever small or great amount of life we have left. Nostalgia allows us to rediscover something of our forgotten future. Psychiatry, which seeks the possible connections between past and future, cannot live without the great works from which it draws.

There are consonances, but also, and perhaps above all, dissonances between the essence of nostalgia and of regret: in the first, we think back to the pain of the things fate kept us from doing, and in the second, we think back to the things we could have done but didn't do. These seems to me to be the time of regret, of the things that might have been done, but weren't.

The past, consideration of the past, changes vertiginously insofar as our emotions change. The past is not an inert, petrified mass, but a chameleonic one: to reflect upon it helps us to see the things that happen today with a wonder that is ceaselessly reborn.

There is nostalgia for our childhood and adolescence, as Dostoevsky says, which opened up in life for us possibilities we were incapable of realizing. We may have nostalgia for the horizons of life, to which our imagination unconsciously aspired although they've never existed. But the expectation that the impossible can become possible never goes away, and is another way of not letting hope die within us.

Nostalgia runs the risk of imprisoning us in an idealized past that refuses to allow us a future, and that immobilizes us in a desert where nothing will ever bloom.

That image I looked back to at the beginning of this story, one of Brentano's most beautiful, which defines madness as the unhappy sister of poetry, seems to me close in its boldness to another of Giorgio Colli, who calls madness the womb of wisdom; and each of these are images of an impossible hope. Great poetry and great novels allow psychology to broaden and expand its knowledge of the infinite horizons of the soul. In Hölderlin, in Gérard de Nerval, in Sylvia Plath, in Robert Walser, madness and poetry flow together in extraordinary creative association, at times incomparable, as Karl Jaspers said, in its painful beauty.

Bibliography

Augustine. *The Confessions of St. Augustine*. Translated by Albert C. Outler. Dover: 2002.

Arieti, Silvano. *Creativity: The Magic Synthesis*. Basic Books: 1980.

Bachmann, Ingeborg. *Werke*. R. Piper Verlag: 1982.

Basaglia, Franco. *Scritti I, 1953-1968*. Einaudi: 1981.

Scritti II, 1968-1980. Einaudi: 1982.

Conferenze brasiliane. Raffaello Cortina: 2000.

Bauman, Zygmunt. *Liquid Fear*. Polity: 2006.

Bernanos, Georges. *Œuvres romanesques*. Bibliothèque de la Pléiade, Gallimard:1961.

Binswanger, Ludwig. *Schizophrenie*. Neske: 1957.

Melancholie und Manie. Neske: 1960.

Binswanger, Ludwig and Aby Warburg. *Die unendliche Heilung: Aby Warburgs Krankengeschichte*. Diaphenes: 2019.

Blanchot, Maurice. *The Infinite Conversation*. Translated by Susan Hansen. University of Minnesota: 1992.

Bleuler, Manfred. *Die schizophrenen Geistesstörungen im Lichte langjähriger Kranken- und Familiengeschichten*. Thieme: 1972.

Borghi, Marco. "Aspetti giuridici e culturali sul tema del contenimento e della contenzione. Forme di contenzione," in *Atti del convegno su Cure e qualità di vita: la contenzione* (Manno, October 11, 2010), pp. 3-6, in manuscript.

Borgna, Eugenio. "L'esperienza poetica di una schizofrenica," in *Rivista sperimentale di Freniatria*, XCV (1971), pp. 844 and ff.

I conflitti del conoscere. Strutture del sapere ed esperienza della follia. Feltrinelli: 1988.

Malinconia. Feltrinelli: 1992.

Come se finisse il mondo. Il senso dell'esperienza schizofrenica. Feltrinelli: 1995.

L'arcipelago delle emozioni. Feltrinelli: 2001.

L'attesa e la Speranza. Feltrinelli: 2005.

Il tempo e la vita. Feltrinelli: 2015.

L'ascolto gentile. Einaudi: 2017.

Le parole che ci salvano. Einaudi: 2017.

La nostalgia ferita. Einaudi: 2018.

Cabibbe, Feruccio. *Matrimonio manicomio.* Moretti & Vitali: 2013.

Campo, Cristina. *The Unforgivable.* Translates by Alex Andriesse. NYR Classics: 2024.

Canetti, Elias. *The Memoirs of Elias Canetti: The Tongue Set Free, The Torch in My Ear, The Play of the Eyes.* Translated by Joachim Neugroschel. FSG: 1999.

The Book Against Death. Translated by Peter Filkins. New Directions: 2024.

Celan, Paul. *Die Gedichte: Neue kommentierte Gesamtausgabe.* Suhrkamp: 2018.

Colli, Giorgio. *La nascita della filosofia.* Adelphi: 1975.

Ricarda Dick (ed): *Else Lasker-Schüler – Franz Marc. Eine Freundschaft in Briefen und Bildern.* Prestel: 2012.

Dickinson, Emily. *The Poems of Emily Dickinson. Variorum Edition.* Belknap: 1998.

Dostoevsky, Fyodor. *The Brothers Karamazov.* Translated by David McDuff. Penguin Classics: 2003.

Elias, Norbert. *The Loneliness of the Dying.* Translated by Edmund Jephcott. Continuum: 2001.

Frances, Allen. *Saving Normal: An Insider's Revolt against Out-of-Control Psychiatric Diagnosis, DSM-5, Big Pharma, and the Medicalization of Ordinary Life.* Mariner Books: 2014.

Gebsattel, Viktor Emil. *Imago Hominis.* Neues Forum: 1964.

Görner, Rüdiger. *Georg Trakl. Dichter im Jahrzehnt der Extreme.* Zsolnay: 2014.

Guardini, Romano. *Vom Sinn der Schwermut.* Arche: 1949.

Heidegger, Martin. *Being and Time.* Translated by Joan Staumbaugh. SUNY: 2010.

Heidegger, Martin. *On the Way to Language*. HarperOne: 1982.

Hillesum, Etty. *An Interrupted Life: The Diaries and Letters from Westerbork 1941–1943*. Picador: 1996.

Hofmannsthal, Hugo von. *Buch der Freunde*. 1922.

Hölderlin, Friedrich. *Poems and Fragments*. Translated by Michael Hamburger. Anvil Press: 2004.

Jaspers, Karl. *Allgemeine Psychopathologie*. Springer: 1959.

Khayat, David. *De larmes et de sang*. Odile Jacob, Paris 2013.

Kierkegaard, Sören. *The Diary of Sören Kierkegaard*. Peter Rhodes, ed. Citadel: 2000.

Kierkegaard, Søren. *The Essential Kierkegaard*. Translated by Howard V. Hong. Princeton University Press: 2000.

Kundera, Milan. *Identity: A Novel*. Translated by Linda Asher. Harper Perennial: 1999.

Lasker-Schüler, Else. *Hebrew Ballads and Other Poems*. Jewish Publication Society: 1980.

Lauter, H., & Meyer, J. E. (1984). "Active Euthanasia Without Consent: Historical Comments on a Current Debate." *Death Education*, 8 (2-3), 89–98.

Leopardi, Giacomo. *Canti*. Translated by Jonathan Galassi. FSG: 2011.

Leopardi, Giacomo. *Zibaldone*. Translated by Michael Caesar et al. FSG: 2015.

Levinas, Emmanuel. *Carnets de captivité et autres inédits*, ed., Rodolphe Calin and Catherine Chalier.

Œuvres 1, Bernard Grasset/IMEC: 2009.

Lungershausen, E. "Sterbehilfe bei psychisch Kranken? Das neue Gesetz in den Niederlanden," in Martin Brüne and Theo Payk (eds), *Sozialdarwinismus, Genetik und Euthanasie*. Wissenschaftliche Verlagsgesellschaft: 2003.

Mann, Thomas. *The Magic Mountain*. Translated by H.T. Lowe-Porter. Knopf: 1955.

Mann, Thomas. *Josef and His Brothers*. Translated by H.T. Lowe-Porter. Knopf: 1983.

Sandor Marai. *Casanova in Bolzano*. Translated by George Szirtes. Knopf: 2005.

Mieli, Paolo. "Il pretesto della pazzia," in *Corriere della Sera*, 12 December 2017.

Minkowski, Eugène. *La schizophrénie*. Payot: 1927.

Lived Time. Translated by Nancy Wetzel. Northwestern University Press: 2019.

Mittner, Ladislao. *Storia della letteratura tedesca. III/2. Dal fine secolo alla sperimentazione (1890-1979)*. Einaudi: 1971.

Montale, Eugenio. *Collected Poems 1920-1954*. Translated by Jonathan Galassi. FSG: 1997.

Morselli, Giovanni Enrico. "Sulla dissociazione mentale," in *Rivista sperimentale di Freniatria*, LIV (1930), pp. 209 ff.

"In tema di schizofrenia," in *Rivista sperimentale di Freniatria*, LV (1931), pp. 3 ff..

L'esistenza psicopatologica, Minerva Medica: 1975.

Nabokov, Vladimir. *Speak, Memory*. Victor Gollancz: 1951.

Pascal, Blaise. *Pensées*. Translated by A.J. Krailsheimer. Penguin Classics: 1995.

Pavese, Cesare. *The Business of Living: Diary 1935–1950*. Translated by Geoffrey Brock. Routledge: 2009.

Plath, Sylvia. *The Collected Poems*. Harper Perennial: 2018.

Porena, Ida. *La verità dell'immagine. Una lettura di Georg Trakl*. Donzelli: 1998.

Pozzi, Antonia. *Poesia che mi guardi*. Sossella: 2010.

Pozzi, Giovanni. *Tacet*. Adelphi: 2013.

Rilke, Rainer Maria. *Letters of Rainer Maria Rilke, 1892-1910*. Translated by. Jane B. Greene and M.D. Herder Norton. Norton: 1969.

Letters to a Young Poet. Translated by Charlie Louth. Penguin Classics: 2018.

The Notebooks of Malte Laurids Brigge. Translated by Michael Hulse. Penguin Classics: 2009.

The Poetry of Rilke. Translated by Edward Snow. North Point Press: 2011.

Rümke, H. C. *Eine blühende Psychiatrie in Gefahr. Ausgewählte Vorträge und Aufsätze.* Springer: 1967.

Saraceno, Benedetto. *Sulla povertà della psichiatria.* DeriveApprodi: 2017.

Schneider, Kurt. *Klinische Psychopathologie.* Thieme:1959.

Schumann, Robert. *The Letters of Robert Schumann.* Translated by Karl Storck and Hannah Bryant. Ulan Press: 2012.

Shakespeare, William. *Macbeth.* Folger Shakespeare Library: 2013.

Slavich, Antonio. *All'ombra dei ciliegi giapponesi. Gorizia: 1961.* Alphabeta, Merano: 2018.

Sozzi, Lionello. *Gli spazi dell'anima.* Bollati Boringhieri: 2011.

Straus, Erwin. *Vom Sinn der Sinne*, Springer: 1956.

Teresa di Lisieux. *Story of a Soul.* Translated by John Brown. ICS Publications: 2005.

Tolstoy, Leo. *Anna Karenina.* Translated by Louise and Aylmer Maude. Wordsworth Classics: 1997.

Trakl, Georg. *Poems and Prose: A Bilingual Edition.* Translated by Alexander Stillmark. Northwestern University Press: 2005.

Walser, Robert. *The Tanners.* Translated by Susan Bernofsky. New Directions: 2009.

Weil, Simone. *An Anthology.* Edited by Siân Miles. Penguin Classics: 2005.

The Notebooks. Translated by Arthur Wills. Routledge and Kegan Paul: 1956.

Weil, Simone. *Waiting for God.* Translated by Emma Crauford. Harper Colophon: 1973.

Weil, Simone. *Intimations of Christianity Among the Ancient Greeks.* Translated by Elisabeth Chase Geissbuhler. Routledge: 1957

Woolf, Virginia. *The Waves.* Penguin Classics: 2019.

Wyrsch, Jakob. *Psychiatrie als offene Wissenschaft.* Haupt: 1969.

VECTORS

DEFINITION
Vectors are not like typical academic monographs. They are aimed at a
more general audience, which might include undergraduate students,
academics working in other fields, practitioners, policymakers, and the
public. They provide a platform for established academic authors to reach
a larger audience than usual, or to speak to new audiences; to deliver
bold new arguments; to write unencumbered by the usual obligations for
referencing; and to be exciting, provocative and even polemical.

ALREADY PUBLISHED:
Massimo Arcangeli, *Genderless Grammar.*
Alberto Lucarelli, *Tradition & Revolution.*
Eugenio Borgna, *Hope and Despair.*
Eugenio Borgna, *Wounded Nostalgia.*
Eugenio Borgna, *The Madness That is Also in Us.*

COMING SOON:
Simone Gozzano, *Consciousness.*

www.ingramcontent.com/pod-product-compliance
Lightning Source LLC
Chambersburg PA
CBHW070812280326
41934CB00012B/3167